FACING EAST

JINGDUAN YANG, M.D., F.A.P.A.
WITH NORMA KAMALI

WM

WILLIAM MORROW
An Imprint of HarperCollinsPublishers

FACING EAST

Ancient
Health and Beauty
Secrets for
the Modern Age

EAST

FACING EAST. Copyright © 2016 by Jingduan Yang. All rights reserved. Printed in the United States of America. No part of this book may be used or reproduced in any manner whatsoever without written permission except in the case of brief quotations embodied in critical articles and reviews. For information address HarperCollins Publishers, 195 Broadway, New York, NY 10007.

HarperCollins books may be purchased for educational, business, or sales promotional use. For information please e-mail the Special Markets Department at SPsales@harpercollins.com.

FIRST EDITION

Designed by Renato Stanisic

Library of Congress Cataloging-in-Publication Data has been applied for.

ISBN 978-0-06-236346-6

16 17 18 19 20   OV/RRD   10 9 8 7 6 5 4 3 2 1

I want to dedicate this book to my father, who envisioned what this world would need today and prepared me for that. And to my patients and colleagues, who constantly prove to me that the ancient wisdom of the East is being rediscovered and appreciated by modern medicine too.

Contents

Part 3: Your Mind, Heart, and Spirit

've always had many passions. Enhancing the lives of women and empowering them in some way have been a big part of my endeavors. My love of fashion design is one of my most obvious passions. But I am also deeply devoted to finding natural, plant-based solutions and products to meet the needs of my clients in the areas of health, wellness, and beauty. I've been committed to this latter pursuit since 2002 when I established the WELLNESS CAFÉ in my flagship store on West Fifty-Sixth Street in New York City, though my wellness journey began long before then.

I credit my earliest health and beauty training to my mother, who I later realized was way ahead of her times. She was a very unconventional woman whose daily life was built around understanding the best practices for maintaining a strong mind and body. She was already juicing, looking closely at the ingredients on labels, taking vitamins, finding a million miracle uses for olive oil, and exercising the Jack LaLanne way. While other mothers were on what I call the *I Love Lucy* diet, consisting of a canned fruit cocktail, a scoop of cottage cheese, and a slice of melba toast, my mother's view was not traditional. Her kitchen looked like a food-test laboratory. There were pots of green herbs all over the place. The windows had shelves with different plants she nurtured and used in our daily meals. She experimented with a wide variety of combinations. The Mediterranean diet was part of our Lebanese heritage, and that added another healthy factor. I never once thought of her ways as being different until I realized other moms were not the same. However, over time, this lifestyle simply became a part of who I am.

My mother was unorthodox in other ways too. I remember her telling me when I was just eleven years old that I should learn how to take care of myself as a woman so I could be free to marry the man I love rather than the man who could best take care of me. I had no idea then how brilliant this statement was. **Life has been a quest to learn to care for myself ever since, not just financially, but physically, emotionally, and spiritually too, which is a lot of what beauty—and this book—is about.** My mother really set me off on a decades-long adventure to find ways to extend and improve the quality of life. Along the way there have been countless discoveries that really do work, many of which I am eager to share with other people, especially women. While women are vulnerable at times, they are also very powerful in the influence they exert over others. They have sway with their friends, their communities, and especially their families—their husband, children, and often their aging parents as well. Because women can change the world exponentially, it is important for me to try to connect to as many of them as possible with as much information about things we can do to be healthier human beings.

We all know the biggest luxury in life is health. And it just so happens that if you are healthy you are also attractive. The two go hand-in-hand. Beauty is not going to endure any other way. We all look our best when we are in good condition. Our skin glows, our hair shines, our face is brighter, even our eyes sparkle more.

For many of us, there is no better incentive to be healthy than to have the best possible quality of life and to spend more time with our loved ones . . . and, of course, to look good too.

I've been in fashion for nearly my whole life. Feeling and looking one's best is an integral part of that culture. So finding people who have knowledge to share about achieving health and beauty is something I have been doing and will do for the rest of my life.

I receive and read at least ten different wellness newsletters every week, so I am aware of how rapidly the medical community's understanding of health and well-being is shifting. Things we once thought were reliable and dependable are in question, and things we thought we'd never do are all of a sudden looking like safe and appealing alternatives. In the midst of all this change, acupuncture and other age-old practices seem to make all the sense in the world. They have withstood the test of time. Various cultures would not have relied on these practices for centuries if they didn't believe they were effective. People simply don't continue to do things that don't work. Timeless style is my approach to fashion, so my search for the best acupuncturist I could find grew from this reasoning.

My interest intensified in 2010 while I was visiting Beijing on business. When my friends in China told me I could enjoy all the benefits of a face-lift naturally through acupuncture, vanity kicked in and I began an extensive search for a qualified doctor who could give me an acupuncture face-lift. I contacted people who were in the know, and there was one name that kept coming up—Dr. Jingduan Yang. Dr. Yang is an international expert in acupuncture and classical forms of Chinese medicine, as well as a specialist in integrative medicine, psychiatry, and human behavior. Although his offices were some distance away—in South Jersey and Philadelphia—I made the commitment to drive two hours to the New Jersey location and back every Thursday to meet with him. The first meeting was eye opening. He explained to me that before I could have an acupuncture face-lift, I needed to know more about acupuncture and that he would decide when I was ready. Immediately I knew I was with someone I could learn from. I asked if I could tape our meetings, and he agreed.

I instantly respected Dr. Yang for his caution. I loved and appreciated his authenticity and sincerity. He was determined to make me feel both informed and safe before proceeding in a world where I had no prior knowledge. I had been to an acupuncturist two or three times in my life before meeting him and sadly the experiences were less than satisfying, which is why I was so adamant about finding someone reliable and well recommended. So it wasn't until Dr. Yang felt I was absolutely ready that we began my treatment. He wanted me to truly comprehend what acupuncture was about, what would happen in the weeks and months ahead, and how I would ultimately be affected by the experience. To be fully renewed on the outside, you must first be renewed on the inside, organ by organ, system by system, function by function. I had a million questions for him and I loved listening to every one of his answers. There is something very comforting about talking with knowledgeable people. It's like reading a great book—one you don't want to end anytime soon.

Naturally, I learned a tremendous amount in those months. I even had opportunities to tour Thomas Jefferson Hospital in Philadelphia, where the integrative medicine department is situated next to the oncology department. So much valuable collaborative research on our immune system and its effect on our cells, particularly cancer cells, is being done there. Because Dr. Yang knew my mother had Parkinson's before she died, he also showed me what he was doing to help treat patients with that disease. It was remarkable how he was able to help reduce their tremors week after week. It was profound to listen to one patient who had progressed from having a weak, shaky, Katharine Hepburn–type tremble to having a vibrant and robust voice once again. The benefits of the integrative medicine Dr. Yang and others are practicing at the teaching hospital are amazing. The key to helping prevent and fight serious disease is keeping our immune system intact. It's about maintaining the balance of our body's own healing energies. This is also the key to achieving the healthy glow I was looking for. **Basically, an acupuncture face-lift is designed to help improve the body's ability to heal itself, regenerating some of our tired and overworked cells in the process.** If we care for our bodies proactively, we can hopefully avoid getting sick and can even slow or reverse the aging process.

I was very fortunate that my search led me to a master who has a great sense of the mind, body, and soul of each patient. Through the historical perspective on Chinese medicine he provides, the ancient tools he uses, and the innate skills he draws upon, Dr. Yang performs a great service for modern times. To this day, the wise counsel, time-honored healing practices, and deep sleep I experience under his care are as valuable to me as any other aspect of the acupuncture face-lift, including the remarkable, revitalizing effect it has on my overall appearance.

I realize that not everyone has access to such an extraordinary practitioner, and those who do may still be hesitant about trying this or other similar techniques without the kind of education and understanding I was afforded beforehand. For these reasons, I encouraged Dr. Yang to write this book and was happy to collaborate with him on it. Together we want to help you learn some of the same things about classical Chinese medicine, acupuncture, acupressure, diet, exercise, seasonality, and sleep that I discovered in advance of my treatment. **This book was designed specifically to introduce you to exercises and practices you can do at home. We've placed an emphasis on acupressure for those of you who would like to prepare for and supplement your acupuncture treatment, as well as for those of you who wish to achieve some of the same rejuvenating effects without needles.** Our goal was to create a practical tool that you could use every day to achieve noticeable results.

I am absolutely thrilled that you picked up this book. While I don't believe that pursuing youth is necessarily a good thing (I am too much of a believer in forward motion for that, and I am comfortable with how I've evolved over time), I think doing all that you can to look and feel good is important. It means you are putting your best face forward every day. You are healthy, fit, fueled by the energy of all you have learned in life so far and empowered with endless potential for the present and future. Attention to your health makes you feel invincible, and people who feel invincible can accomplish anything.

As you read this book, know that I wish the same for you as my mother wished for me: that the wisdom shared here will help you enjoy a quality of life to the last day—a *beautiful* quality of life where you can look, feel, and *be* your very best. I also wish that you will have as enriching an experience learning and practicing what Dr. Yang teaches about health, wellness, and beauty as I did. So here's to an invincible future!

—Norma Kamali

When I was a little boy growing up in Hefei, a small town in China's Anhui Province, I never could have imagined a world as overrun with anti-aging treatments as the one we live in today. A world filled with so many lotions, serums, formulas, and procedures—all promising "supple, radiant, youthful skin"; "plumper, dewy lips"; "voluminous hair"; "lustrous lashes and brows"; and "sparkling white teeth." A world where new cosmetic products and techniques are introduced almost daily, but with mixed and largely superficial results. While the options can be overwhelming, all too often the results are underwhelming—and not particularly long-lasting.

I also never imagined that I would become a practitioner of classical Chinese medicine. This is such an important legacy in my culture that it wasn't likely that my father—a fourth-generation practitioner—would pass it down to the youngest of his eight children. It's actually customary to teach this art and science to your firstborn male child, as he is the one who carries the family lineage. But I became the exception to this rule as an act of preservation—*my* preservation. I was raised during the Great Cultural Revolution. My oldest brother was sent to the countryside to be re-educated by Mao's farmers, as all of the teenagers were at that time. He never had a chance to learn classical Chinese medicine, so my father taught these skills to me instead. Because I was a somewhat spoiled daydreamer who mostly loved to play and eat, he was concerned that I'd never survive the harsh conditions on the farms if I were sent there too. So he prepared me to become what was called a *barefoot doctor*—a practitioner who tended to the illnesses of the workers in the flooded wheat paddies of Southern China with nothing more than a box of needles and some basic herbs. He thought I might at least be fed enough to get by if I was useful to the farmers in this way. So at the age of thirteen I began my training with him by reading textbooks on Chinese medicine. Most of these original source books were written in the ancient Chinese language. I also began practicing how to locate acupuncture points and insert and manipulate needles on straw papers and on myself.

Although I was never sent to the farms, because the Great Cultural Revolution ended after Mao's death in the late 1970s, that early education became the foundation of my nearly four-decade-long study and practice of classical Chinese medicine. I was really very lucky to have had that experience. So much of the knowledge and the special skills those texts taught me have been lost over the years. And some of these traditional teachings were modified first by China's communist ideology and later by the increased use of Western medicine in the East.

You could also add studying *modern* medicine on four different continents with some of the most respected doctors in their fields to the growing list of things I never imagined I would do. After a higher education system in China resumed, I attended one of China's top modern medical schools—the Fourth Military Medical University in Xi'an City, Shaanxi. I later continued my studies at the WHO Collaborating Centre for Research and Training in Mental Health in Shanghai. I also became one of the first students to study outside of China on an exchange program with the University of Sydney in Australia and to complete a research fellowship at Oxford University in England.

I specialized in neurology and psychiatry because I was especially intrigued by the way the mind-body connection affects an individual's physical, mental, and spiritual health. It was a fascination that developed when I was very young as I watched my father care for some of the psychiatric patients he treated. It wasn't until much later that I would delve into how much the mind-body connection affects beauty as well.

The radically different medical systems I was learning—Chinese and Western medicine—sometimes clashed with and contradicted each other, but I gradually began to appreciate their similarities and differences. By the time I came to the United States, I was fluent in ancient and modern, Eastern and Western, physical and emotional, as well as energetic and biochemical medicine. I completed my residency at Thomas Jefferson University in Philadelphia and a two-year-long integrative medicine fellowship at the University of Arizona before founding the Tao Institute of Mind and Body Medicine.

But the events I *really* never anticipated were meeting the force of nature known as Norma Kamali . . . and deciding to collaborate with her on this book. This iconic fashion designer (who, by the way, was fit, striking, and full of life to begin with) first came to me as a patient, but her interest in bringing relevant health and beauty knowledge to the public quickly endeared her to me as a friend too. She asked me so many astute questions about how to achieve and preserve complete wellness that it wasn't long before I realized that we were on parallel missions. Through my practice, I share some of classical Chinese medicine's oldest and most hidden secrets with others as a way of helping them achieve the kind of lasting health on the inside that radiates as enduring beauty on the outside. **In many ways you could say that I am offering my patients a natural health lift that results in a natural face-lift too!**

Norma's and my many sessions together reminded me of passages right out of a book I've studied consistently from the time my father first introduced me to it. The book I am referring to is a massive two-volume tome that was written in the ancient Chinese language more than 2,500 years ago. It is called *Huang Di Nei Jing* (translated as *The Yellow Emperor's Classic Inner Canon*). The book follows a dialogue—actually, a series of questions and answers—between an extremely inquisitive emperor and several of his most knowledgeable health advisors. Norma's curiosity was just like the emperor's, and because I had read and referred to this work so often over the years, my answers sounded very much like those of the advisors, complemented, of course, by my many studies since then.

As I told Norma, what makes this ancient text—and the Chinese medical practice derived from it—so exceptional is that *it presents a far more comprehensive view of the workings of the human body than anything that has been written since*. It unveils a *complete* medical system for the diagnosis and prevention of disease and the preservation of health and life. Unlike modern Western medicine, which approaches health from a mostly structural and biochemical perspective, this system visualizes and explains every human function on those two levels *and* on the bioenergetic and spiritual levels. In the process it reveals details about the mind-body connection that can help heal, restore, and maintain us naturally on a molecular level, leaving us feeling and looking more youthful and vibrant than ever.

Because there was no documentation as to how this complete medical system was developed, some people question whether *Huang Di Nei Jing* was indeed written by the best minds in China at the time. There are some who hypothesize that members of a preexisting, advanced civilization—survivors perhaps of some catastrophic event—gifted this comprehensive life-knowledge to the Chinese people through a series of briefings that were then compiled into this miraculous source book. When you think of the time, funding, research, and trial testing that even the smallest breakthroughs in modern medicine require, this hypothesis seems more than plausible. If these folks are right, why wouldn't we consider following advice from a knowledge base greater than our own?

The more Norma and I talked, the more we realized how many people had the same questions she did—and how many people would appreciate knowing some of the secrets *Huang Di Nei Jing* contained, especially those that pertained to maintaining enduring beauty. It also became apparent that my unexpected and varied life experiences, which bridged such different sciences, cultures, and languages, made me uniquely prepared to help decode the book's many revelations for this new and eager audience and to present it in a manner that fits today's varied needs and rich lifestyles.

Maybe when you were younger there were things you couldn't imagine either. Perhaps you thought you'd never need a little help around the eyes, under the chin, or around the middle. That your mental, physical, emotional, and spiritual health could never impact your beauty as much as it does now. Or that you'd never find practical, natural, and long-lasting solutions to your health and beauty challenges. But as someone who was led to this point in life and career by a long string of surprises, I am here to encourage you to be open to the pleasant surprises ahead for you too.

Having studied and practiced both classical Chinese medicine and modern Western medicine so extensively, I genuinely believe that classical Chinese medicine is like the wise elder statesman, worthy of our reverence and attention, while modern medicine is more like a young whippersnapper racing to catch up. As health care in America continues to grapple with its many problems; as people turn to an increasing number of alternative treatments for the challenges they face; as they seek quick cosmetic fixes for more complex issues; and as modern medicine's findings slowly but surely corroborate and validate the truths revealed in ancient Chinese texts, I feel compelled to share these life-altering practices with you in terms you can readily understand and apply to your total health and beauty regimen.

It is not worth the wait of another two millennia for modern medicine to finally arrive at the same conclusions these time-honored texts offer us. We should all be able to rejuvenate, heal, and enjoy a fuller, more visible vitality *now*. The truly integrative approach to mind, body, and spiritual well-being that was revealed to the Chinese culture centuries ago can and should be applied to all cultures today. I have written *Facing East* in collaboration with Norma Kamali, using an accessible question-and-answer format much like the book that inspired this one, for exactly this reason.

As you turn the pages, you will find easy, practical, day-to-day steps you can take to improve all aspects of your inner and outer well-being—steps drawn from a wisdom that has remained hidden and dormant for too long.

But before we begin, it is important to note that *Facing East* is not a consultation, diagnostic, or treatment book, nor can it possibly exhaust all that *Huang Di Nei Jing* has to say. Think of it more as a mirror that reflects the connections between the internal you and the perceptible you, so that you can manage your overall health better and emanate the kind of individual beauty we all wish to.

I sincerely hope that the age-old truths you find on these pages will renew, revive, sustain, and please you for many years to come.

—Jingduan Yang, M.D., F.A.P.A.

1

Your Energy

1

Testing, Testing, 1, 2, 3

WHAT IS YOUR BODY TELLING YOU?

Because of the way I was raised and the way I presently care for my body, I am very attuned to the messages it sends me. I can tell when something is off by even a little bit and can make adjustments to my diet, exercise, or sleep routine right away to help get back on track. I don't like to take medication—even antibiotics—and when I have to, I do it kicking and screaming. I am aware, however, that I am just one of many different types of patients. Some people blatantly ignore their body's signals, dismissing the symptoms they are experiencing as normal or as something they just have to tolerate. Other people's habits actually mask their body's messages. I know this because for a brief period in my late twenties I casually smoked cigarettes, ate bacon cheeseburgers, and drank Coca-Cola. While I *never* did recreational drugs and I don't like alcohol all that much, I indulged in candy a lot back then too. One night during that unusual period in my life, I woke up and smelled tobacco every-where. It made me so sick I never smoked again. It was as if some other force said to me, "You're not going to smoke anymore," because I quit instantly. I had a similar experience with coffee at the time. I'm not quite sure how or why I ever fell into that pattern, but after my senses returned and I resumed the lifestyle I have now, I realized just how much unhealthy choices can prevent us from having a real dialogue with our body. How could I not know that drinking too much caffeine was what made me sneeze eleven times in a row?!

For a lot of people who tend to mask messages in this way, seeing their doctor at least once a year is how they check in with their body. People are like this with beauty issues as well. Some only take care of their skin when there are breakouts, or when wrinkles first appear, while others have been attentive since they were teens. **So my first question for Dr. Yang is: No matter what type of patient we are, no matter what brought us to this book, no matter how general or specific our reasons are for seeking your guidance, how do we use what we find in these pages as proactively as possible?**

Norma's first question gets right to the heart of this book. I really want to engage patients in a different way of communicating with their bodies—and with their doctors—for the sake of their overall health, well-being, and countenance.

In Western culture, when you see your doctor for an annual physical, he or she will most likely chat with you for a few minutes to see if anything major is going on in your life. Then they will proceed to check your heart, lungs, head, neck, and abdomen for the development of any structural abnormalities. They will also look at your blood count, run a urinalysis, and perform some other routine tests checking the biochemical status of your metabolism, hormones, organ functions, and blood cells, noting any differences from your last visit. They are *looking for problems* with the intent of addressing them before they progress any further.

Similarly, when you visit your doctor with a particular set of symptoms or a specific concern, you are there largely because you fear that you may have *found a problem* and you want to stop it in its tracks. In both contexts, you and your doctor have a laser-like focus on what may go wrong—if it hasn't already gone wrong.

But to subscribe to the theories of Chinese medicine and to use this book effectively, you must embrace the idea that maintaining good health and beauty is not necessarily

about catching problems in time. It is about actively cultivating good health so problems don't develop in the first place. It is also about being in touch with your body on a much deeper level than just noticing symptoms when they first appear.

While it's encouraging to see that some Western doctors are moving away from a troubleshooting approach and are administering far better preventative care, they are still a long way from knowing the human condition as well as practitioners of Chinese medicine comprehend it. They consistently fail to check one of the most important determinants of how well we are functioning because it simply isn't within their philosophy, scope, or study. This determinant can be found in our *energy level*.

If you have ever engaged in energy-based therapies such as Reiki, qigong, meditation, or acupuncture, then you know how effective attending to your energy can be. Yet despite the consistent good health of people who incorporate these therapies into their lives and the remarkable recoveries of people who have turned to them in crisis, there are still many skeptics out there—particularly in the modern-medicine community—who just can't imagine how such results are possible.

In some ways their reactions are understandable because energy is not something that we can easily see. But what they must understand is that energy is just like the air we breathe. We live in it and it lives in us. If we condition ourselves properly, we can feel the difference when its quality and quantity change.

Practitioners of traditional Chinese medicine have been attuned to human energy and have successfully worked with it for centuries as a means of restoring and retaining good health. **We call this energy Q**i (pronounced "chi").

In everyday living, and certainly in clinical practice, we encounter *Qi* all the time. Whenever you hear people say things such as "I'm so tired," "I feel nauseous," "My head is exploding," "I'm so pissed off," "My hands and feet are always so cold," or "I'm having hot flashes and am sweating a lot," what they are describing is the imbalance or disruption of the energy inside them.

The challenge for modern medicine is that it has yet to *visualize* human energy the way Chinese medicine has. Modern medicine can only measure some of our energy's activity through EKGs, ENGs, EMGs, and EEGs, whereas ancient Chinese medicine actually provides detailed descriptions and a complete map of our energetic anatomy, physiology, and pathophysiology. We know exactly how our energies travel through the body, in the same way that we all know how blood flows through veins, arteries, and capillaries. We can track our energies' movement through defined channels we call *Jing Luo*, often translated as "meridians." We know which organs these energies connect with and what function they serve along their route. We see this dimension of the human condition *in addition* to what modern medicine is capable of seeing.

By looking exclusively at the structural and biochemical aspects of health, modern medicine sees only a portion of your complete wellness picture. **It can only identify health problems when your condition has worsened to the point where those problems are evident and can be measured.** By contrast, Chinese medicine teaches us that health issues don't just occur overnight. They begin within the deeper energetic levels of our body. Becoming attuned to your energy levels and learning to keep them in balance is how you avoid the development of disease and how you truly maintain good health inside and out.

To help you attain greater benefit from the health and beauty tips offered throughout this book, and from the medical care you seek for yourself as you move forward in life, I've included a modified version of a questionnaire developed and used regularly in China by Dr. Qi Wang, an expert in this field. I ask every patient who comes to see me in my clinic to complete the questionnaire during their first visit, as it provides a very valuable overview of their energetic constitution based on the theories of ancient Chinese medicine. It helps determine if their energy tends to be too Cool, too Warm, too Damp, too Dry, too Deficient, and if it's moving freely in the right direction or not circulating well enough.

Please note that this version of the questionnaire requires only yes or no answers to help make scoring it easier; however, if you wish to complete the original, more nuanced version, it can be found in the appendix of this book along with detailed instructions on how to tally the results.

As you will see, the questionnaire is broken down into eight parts. Each is designed to address a different type of energy imbalance. The first seven sets of questions are used to measure for anomalies in specific types of energies. The final set of questions helps to determine if the patient's overall energy is well balanced. In each of the first seven sections, if the majority of your answers are no, your energy in that regard is very likely to be well balanced. If your responses are more frequently yes, you will likely need to attend to those energies more carefully. Discovering your energetic constitution in this way can give you a better sense of which practices described in this book are most relevant and have the greatest potential to benefit you. It will also help you take the first step in having that meaningful, productive, and continual conversation with your body that we believe is so crucial to your health, well-being, and beauty.

Bear in mind that your energetic constitution changes over time, especially if you are exposed to greater environmental, emotional, psychological, and physical stressors—or on the positive side, if you have taken significant measures to live a healthier lifestyle. For this reason, I encourage my patients to revisit this useful tool from time to time to see how their energies are faring at any given moment. A digital copy of the questionnaire lives on my website at www.jdyangmd.com for repeated access. I also encourage you to have a complete evaluation of your energy by a practitioner of classical Chinese medicine near you. Chapter 5 includes tips on how to find one who can meet your needs.

Are you ready and excited to learn more about your personal energetic health? If so, let's get started. And please remember that *all answers should reflect your experience and feelings within the past twelve months.*

YANG DEFICIENCY

QUESTIONS	YES	NO
1. Do your hands or feet ever feel cold?		
2. Are your stomach/abdomen, back, lower back, or knees sensitive to the cold?		
3. Do you wear more clothing than other people to keep warm because you are very sensitive to cold temperatures?		
4. Are you less tolerant of cold temperatures than others? (i.e., less tolerant of the winter, air-conditioning, or fans)?		
5. Are you prone to catching colds more than others or to retaining water in your body?		
6. Do you feel uncomfortable when you eat cold food or drink cold beverages? Or do you have an aversion to cold food and beverages?		
7. After you are exposed to the cold or have cold food or beverages, do you tend to develop diarrhea?		

YIN DEFICIENCY

QUESTIONS	YES	NO
1. Do you ever feel hot on your palms or on the soles of your feet?		
2. Do your face and body feel feverish?		
3. Do your skin and lips feel dry?		
4. Are your lips naturally redder than others' lips?		
5. Are you easily constipated or do you have dry stools?		
6. Is your face flushed or reddish in color?		
7. Do you have a dry mouth or dry eyes?		
8. Do you sweat easily upon mild exertion, or do you sweat at night?		

QI DEFICIENCY

QUESTIONS	YES	NO
1. Are you easily tired?		
2. Do you experience shortness of breath or have difficulty catching your breath?		
3. Do you get heart palpitations easily?		
4. Do you get light-headed or dizzy when you stand up?		
5. Do you catch cold more often than others?		
6. Do you prefer being silent to talking?		
7. Is your voice weak when you are speaking?		
8. Do you sweat spontaneously or with only mild exertion?		

DAMPNESS AND PHLEGM

QUESTIONS	YES	NO
1. Do you feel congestion in your chest and are you bloated or full in your abdominal region?		
2. Do you feel heaviness throughout your entire body and limbs?		
3. Do you have a lot of belly fat?		
4. Do you have an oily secretion on your forehead?		
5. Are your upper eyelids swollen?		
6. Do you have a sticky feeling in your mouth?		
7. Do you have a lot of phlegm, and does it always make you feel as if your throat is being blocked?		
8. Do you have a thick, greasy coating on your tongue?		

DAMPNESS AND HEAT

QUESTIONS	YES	NO
1. Do your face and nose feel greasy or look luminous due to excessive oil secretion?		
2. Do you develop acne and boils easily?		
3. Do you have a bitter or other peculiar taste in your mouth?		
4. Do you feel as if your stool is sticky and hard to eliminate completely?		
5. Do you have a burning sensation when you urinate? Is your urine a dark yellow color?		
6. For women: Is your vaginal discharge a yellow color?		
7. For men: Do you feel wet or damp on your scrotum?		

BLOOD STASIS

QUESTIONS	YES	NO
1. Do you have signs of purple petechia (bleeding under the skin)?		
2. Do you have visible capillaries on your cheeks?		
3. Do you have pain anywhere on your body?		
4. Does your facial coloring appear dark or gloomy? Are you prone to having chloasma (dark brown spots) on your face?		
5. Are you prone to having black circles around your eyes?		
6. Do you tend to be forgetful?		
7. Is your natural lip color purplish?		

SENSITIVITIES

QUESTIONS	YES	NO
1. Do you sneeze even when you do not have a cold?		
2. Do you have nasal congestion and a runny nose even when you do not have a cold?		
3. Do you cough or wheeze in reaction to the change of seasons and climate or in reaction to fragrances?		
4. Do you tend to be allergic to medicines, foods, odors, pollen, or season and climate changes?		
5. Do you have urticaria (hives or raised light red bumps) on your skin?		
6. Do you have purpura (purplish red discoloration) on your skin due to allergies?		
7. Does your skin look scraped when you scratch it?		

QI STAGNATION

QUESTIONS	YES	NO
1. Do you feel unhappy?		
2. Do you easily feel nervous or anxious?		
3. Are you overly sentimental and emotionally fragile?		
4. Do you feel scared or frightened?		
5. Do you have congestion or pain in your breast or hypochondriac area (the region just above your abdomen)?		
6. Do you sigh for no apparent reason?		
7. Do you feel something in your throat that you cannot spit up?		

BALANCED QI

QUESTIONS	YES	NO
1. Are you energetic?		
2. Are you prone to feeling fatigued?		
3. Is your voice weak when you are speaking?		
4. Do you feel unhappy?		
5. Is your body more sensitive to cold temperatures than others (i.e., sensitive to the winter, air-conditioning, or fans)?		
6. Do you adapt well to changes in natural or social environments?		
7. Do you have insomnia?		
8. Are you forgetful?		

Here are a few more post-survey questions for you to consider: Were you at all surprised by your answers? Or were you already somewhat aware of your body's reactions? Did you see any patterns forming? Do you now have greater confidence in your listening abilities? Or did you learn that they need some work as well?

WHAT ALL OF THIS MEANS FOR YOU

Even without knowing much about Chinese medicine, you can intuit from the nature of the questions that when one's cold energy or *Yin Qi is deficient*, one's warm energy or *Yang Qi* is in relative excess. Patients with this deficiency will often have a dry mouth, nose, and throat, and will feel heat in their palms and the bottoms of their feet. They also tend to favor cold drinks, and suffer from constipation, insomnia, anxiety, restlessness, and hyperactivity. In addition, they may have a dry, red tongue and a rapid, thin pulse. Their skin, lips, and eyes dehydrate easily and their faces—particularly their cheeks—often appear flushed. Because of their general sensitivity to dryness and heat, summer and fall are tough seasons for them. Menopausal women typically have *Yin* Deficiency syndrome.

When one's warm energy or *Yang Qi* **is deficient,** one's cool energy or *Yin Qi* is in relative excess. Such people may experience an increased sensation of cold, especially in the hands and feet. Other symptoms include diarrhea, slow metabolism, water retention, low blood pressure, and feelings of fatigue. They also tend to have a light-colored, swollen tongue and a deep and slow pulse. Their facial complexion is often pale, their eyes tend to be puffy or to have bags beneath them, and they also experience nasal congestion with or without a runny nose. Because they are generally sensitive to Cold, Wind, and Damp energy, winter and fall are tough seasons for them.

When one's overall energy or **overall Qi is deficient,** one tends to feel easily tired and experience shortness of breath upon mild exertion. Such people may also sweat spontaneously and have a soft, low voice and a puffy, light-red colored tongue with tooth marks along the sides. Their muscles grow loose and weak and their metabolism slows. They catch cold easily and tend to have a dull facial complexion, dark circles around their eyes, and a puffy face as well. Because they are generally sensitive to Wind, Cold, Damp, and Heat energy, each of the seasons pose specific challenges for them.

When one's energy or *Qi* **is Damp and Phlegmy,** one tends to be overweight, especially in the belly. Such people may also have thick saliva and a greasy tongue coating. This condition can lead to an increase in mucus throughout the respiratory system, heavy sweating, a craving for sweets and fatty foods, and an overall sensitivity to Damp energy. They tend to experience heaviness in their chests and are susceptible to stroke, diabetes, and heart disease. They are also prone to having an oily face, swollen lips, baggy eyes, and nasal congestion.

When one's energy or *Qi* **is Damp and Overheated,** it can lead to swollen joints, fatigue, and an overall heaviness in the body; a red tongue with a thick, yellowish coating; and a slippery, rapid pulse. People with this constitution tend to have a dry mouth with a bitter taste, bad breath, sinusitis with congestion and yellow discharge, constipation, irritability and agitation, as well as bowel and bladder infections. Females also tend to have more vaginal discharge while males are prone to having a wet and itchy scrotum. Facial acne, a ruddy complexion with a greasy film, or jaundiced eyes are also indications of this constitution.

When one's energy or *Qi* **causes Blood Stasis,** one tends to suffer from sharp and severe pain in the location where the stagnation is occurring. For women, migraines, more pronounced symptoms of PMS, and mood changes will frequently result. Their faces and overall complexions will also bear signs, including purple spots. They tend to have gloomy, dark red lips, a dark red nose, and a dark red tongue also marked by purple spots. The veins underneath their tongue may be congested as well.

When one's energy or *Qi* **is sensitive,** one is prone to having allergies. It can sometimes indicate that one's *Qi* is moving in the wrong direction and that toxins are not being expelled properly. In these instances, people have breakouts as their body tries to emit toxins through the pores in their skin or through other means. They are also apt to have a puffy red face and a red runny nose.

Lastly, when one's *Qi* **is stagnant,** one's energy is not moving about freely enough. Such people may experience pain, indigestion, depression, irritable bowels and bladder, agitation, and anxiety. This *Qi* condition indicates the possibility of a blockage in one's system. *Qi,* under these circumstances, can become misdirected. When that happens, people may feel nauseous, they may vomit, or they may feel short of breath, wheeze, or cough. Those with this constitution also tend to have a dull pallor to their face or visible capillaries on their nose and cheeks. Occasionally the muscles around the jaw may tighten, making it difficult to chew, yawn, or talk, as happens to patients with TMJ (temporomandibular joint dysfunction).

Do one or more of these energetic conditions sound familiar to you? (Yes, you can experience several of them at once!) If so, rest assured that throughout this book, you will find a wide range of simple practices—both physical and emotional— that can be implemented to help you. As you adopt some of them, be sure to notice how your outward appearance benefits too!

EASY THINGS YOU CAN *INSTANTLY* DO TO HELP BALANCE YOUR ENERGY

No matter what your energetic constitution is at this moment in time, here are some general things you can do immediately to improve your energy flow and balance!

Eat foods with a variety of colors and tastes: Different foods provide different nutritional values as well as specific types of energy to the body. Eating the same kinds of food over and over again will not only produce deficits in nutrition, but can also cause you to develop sensitivities to those foods, generating inflammation and creating blockages and deficiency in your essential energy flow. This can happen when foods that are touted as *superfoods* rise in popularity—like the current favorite, kale. It's important to bear in mind that even eating healthy, favorable foods in excess can have the opposite of the desired effect. More of a good thing is not always better. Trust in the motto that everything should be enjoyed in moderation.

Banish ice-cold foods and drinks from your table: Cold beverages, soups, and sadly—though not surprisingly—gelato, frozen yogurt, and ice cream constrict the pathways through which energy travels, and therefore, prevent the flow of energy to key organs. They also constrict the flow of blood through your arteries and vessels. Because the Stomach and Intestines need large supplies of both energy and blood to properly digest food, consuming cold foods and beverages can often lead to indigestion, acid reflux, an inefficient metabolism, and overall lethargy.

Protect your extremities from chilling winds: Wind is the energy that allows Cold to invade the body, particularly around the joints where major energy points are located. It is important to remember this in the springtime when wind is prevalent and the anticipation of warmer weather before it actually arrives can sometimes leave us underdressed. Much in the way that eating cold foods and drinking cold beverages causes the constriction of your energy meridians, the same is true when cold air enters the body. Even modern medicine recognizes that a change in weather can greatly affect you, especially if you have conditions such as Raynaud's syndrome or rheumatoid arthritis. So in addition to dressing to protect yourself from the wind when you are outdoors, also be aware of the flow of air in your home or office as it enters through open windows and is circulated by fans and/or air conditioners. Block or stay clear of any other drafts you detect in the space around you. This applies when you are in restaurants and other public places too. If, despite your best efforts, Wind *Qi* does permit Cold

15

to enter your body, causing the meridians to constrict and arthritic pain, general muscle ache, a stiff neck, tension headaches, or chills and fever to manifest, massage the Gallbladder 20 acupuncture point per the illustration shown here.

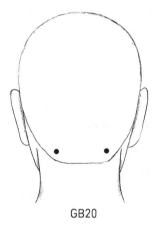

GB20

You can find the Gallbladder 20 point in the large hollows at the base of your skull bone between the trapezius and sternocleidomastoid muscles. Use your thumbs to press on these points while you spread your fingers on the sides of your head. Apply gradual and firm pressure with your fingers into the center of your scalp. Take long and deep breaths, breathing in when you release the pressure and breathing out when you apply the pressure.

This is an effective way to disperse Wind *Qi* from your body and get some fast relief!

Get up and exercise your Qi: Taking a half-hour walk, especially after meals, and breathing deeply as you go will work wonders for increasing your energy flow.

Also, if you have a sedentary job and are seated at a desk for long periods of time, be sure to stand and move about at least once an hour. Stretching exercises will keep your energy circulating as well.

It helps to engage in energy-based activities too. Try meditation, tai chi, yoga, or qigong. Or treat yourself to an acupuncture session or a massage on a more regular basis.

What All of This Means for You

Norma Muses on Conversations with Your Body

Communication is the key to all healthy relationships, so it stands to reason that if you want to have a beautiful and healthy relationship with your body, you will learn to listen to it the same way you listen to those you love. You'll also learn to talk to your doctor or practitioner about what you hear when you are in dialogue with your body. While all of this requires a concerted effort on your part initially, I promise you, over time you won't even realize you're doing it constantly. It will become second nature to you. You'll know instantly what that tickle in your throat or that dry cough is telling you the same way you completely understand the unspoken messages your loved one is sending with a certain look. You will also move quickly to remedy the situation, avoiding the offending food or fragrance or other environmental irritant. Until you get to that point of understanding every nuance, the basic energy-balancing suggestions in this chapter and the test Dr. Yang has supplied to help you figure out your energetic constitution can help you start understanding all those messages better. I always thought that timing your annual mammogram to an event you will remember was a smart, practical, and caring thing to do for yourself. So you might want to follow this example and schedule your energy test at the same time. Plan to take it each year on your birthday when you make your other wellness visits. Or an even better idea is to take the test every time you get your haircut or when you clean out your closet and refresh your wardrobe with the change of seasons. These occasions provide easy enough reminders because you are already focused on giving yourself a lift. Why not make it a health lift? I think that once you're more aware, you'll also be more inclined to use positive practices. It may surprise you at first, but when you listen more attentively to your body, you will very likely discover what a good conversationalist it can be.

2

The Essence of Chinese Medicine

DEMYSTIFYING ITS FOUNDATIONAL THEORIES

Discovering that we have an energetic constitution is fascinating, but it raises a lot of other questions. We all know that the planet and the universe emit and exchange energy all the time. The weather and events like earthquakes and volcanic eruptions are reminders of that. The way energy is harnessed from wind, water, the sun, and parts of the earth to fuel our lifestyle is proof as well. **But our sense of where our own internal energy comes from is more vague than that.** We comment on how much or how little energy we have all the time so we are at least subliminally aware of it as an entity. We even schedule spa appointments to help restore our energy when we feel it's depleted. We have a sense that the phases of the moon affect us too. But these are more intuitive than knowledgeable responses to the energetic shifts in our body. **Dr. Yang, now that we know energy exists inside of us in a very real and formal way—not just a figurative one—can you tell us where this energy comes from? How it changes within our bodies? How we can conserve it . . . and, if it is deficient, how we can replenish it?**

These are all great questions. I especially like how Norma talked about intuitively knowing what our energy is saying to us. In addition to teaching you how to periodically determine your overall energetic constitution, **one of my major goals is to teach you how to consciously use and supplement your energy.**

I'm also glad that spa treatments were mentioned, because while I enjoy them as much as the next person, it's important to note that spa treatments are just one small part of a complete wellness plan. Too many people are lulled into thinking they've addressed their energy needs because they've had a "Hands-on, Chin-ease Meridian Massage" or they've enjoyed a half-hour "Herbs of the Orient Aroma-Therapy" session. When you sample a spa's menu options without a deeper understanding of how *holistic* Chinese medicine really is, it's as if you're choosing to treat your depleted energy with just a Band-Aid instead of the many other remedies available to you in nature's first-aid kit. Spa offerings certainly make us feel good, but they don't necessarily heal us. Learning all about how your energy works will help you make better health and beauty choices on spa days, and on every other day of the year too. It will also make a huge difference in how you look and feel for decades to come, not just how you look and feel in the moment.

To help you get a broader picture of your internal energies, I've identified some of the most important terms and concepts you need to know and have included them in the following quick primer.

ENERGY PRIMER

You may encounter some words here that you are already familiar with, but it is important to read more about them anyway. Some of their meanings were lost in translation when they were first introduced to the West. A new understanding can make a world of difference in your self-care. As you return to take the test provided in chapter 1 several months from now, these definitions will also help provide a deeper understanding of the results.

While there is no quiz at the end of this chapter, how long you live and how youthful you still look in your autumn years will determine whether you've passed the test of time!

JING

The essence of *Qi* is something called *Jing*. You could say *Jing* is what *Qi* is comprised of—the quintessential matter that gives it its life-sustaining qualities. *Jing* is what helps repair whatever needs fixing in your body. *Jing* actually exists in two forms, both of which are stored in the Kidneys, where *Qi* returns to be replenished.

PRENATAL JING

The first form of this essence is known as *Prenatal Jing*. It is the finite quantity of vitality we are all born with. It is passed along to us from our parents at the time of our conception, and we in turn pass some of it along to our offspring during reproduction. How respectfully we use this inherited reserve of energy determines our longevity—how quickly or how slowly we age. Since it must last us a lifetime, and since it ensures the health of our progeny, it should be maintained, conserved, and used wisely.

POSTNATAL JING

The second form of *Qi*'s essence is called *Postnatal Jing,* and it is intended to support our daily use of *Qi* and supplement our *Prenatal Jing*. It is derived from the foods we eat and the air we breathe. When both forms of *Jing*—our *Prenatal* and *Postnatal Jing*—are exhausted, we can no longer sustain the life force within us and, simply put, we die.

QI

As I've already mentioned, *Qi* is what traditional Chinese medicine calls the vital energy that exists within us. It is the life force that propels and keeps everything inside us alive and in motion. But it is also a form of energy that exists outside of us. It is at the root of every function in the human body *and* in the universe.

SHEN

Another important kind of energy traveling inside your body is a *spiritual* energy that Chinese medicine calls *Shen*. *Shen*, *Qi*, and *Jing* are considered the three treasures that enable life. *Shen* is behind consciousness, emotions, thought, sensory and motor function, inspiration, and creativity. It's a positive energy that manifests outwardly as a certain kind of spark or radiance—a love or zest for life. At other times it projects as a calm, peaceful compatibility—a belonging or oneness with everything natural around us. It is also sometimes said that *Shen* is responsible for the intangible beauty we sense when we are around people who feature-for-feature may not possess our culture's classic beauty ideals, but are still undeniably attractive to us.

In the same way that *Jing* (essence) is stored in the Kidneys, *Shen* is stored in the Heart.

Chinese medicine holds the view that whatever exists in nature exists in us and whatever exists in us is reflected in nature. If we are part of the universe and we have a heart and mind, then surely the universe has a heart and mind too. When *Shen* is optimal, the heart and mind of the universe and the heart and mind of the body are one.

MERIDIANS

Now here's one of the most amazing things about our energy: As if it is nature's very own time-released youth capsule, *Qi* circulates throughout our body along the invisible channels I mentioned before called *Jing Luo*, or meridians, delivering vital energy that rejuvenates, repairs, and nourishes virtually every part of us on a regular basis. The meridian system is an enormously complicated one in which each specific channel is named after one of the organ systems that serve the body's specific functions. These organ systems are able to fulfill their function delivering *Jing*, *Qi*, *Shen*, fluid, and blood to their destinations through the meridians. These meridians run parallel to our nervous, cardiovascular, hormonal, and blood systems. The next figure illustrates the Liver Meridian. For ease of reference you will find in the appendix similar illustrations for each of the meridians we discuss.

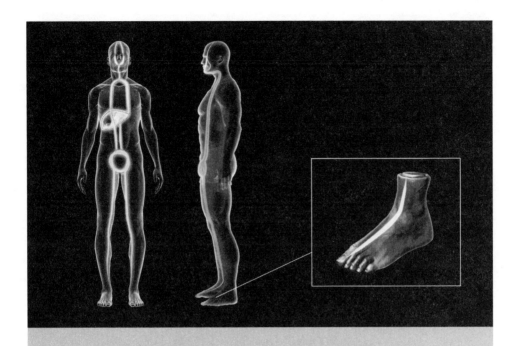

As you can see, *Qi* travels in the meridians in circuits. It concentrates on specific organs at specific times. If all is progressing smoothly, the stops *Qi* makes along these channels can be timed as follows:

Gallbladder	11 P.M.–1 A.M.
Liver	1 A.M.–3 A.M.
Lungs	3 A.M.–5 A.M.
Large Intestine	5 A.M.–7 A.M.
Stomach	7 A.M.–9 A.M.
Spleen	9 A.M.–11 A.M.
Heart	11 A.M.–1 P.M.
Small Intestine	1 P.M.–3 P.M.
Urinary Bladder	3 P.M.–5 P.M.
Kidneys	5 P.M.–7 P.M.
Pericardium	7 P.M.–9 P.M.
Triple Burner*	9 P.M.–11 P.M.

*This term, which is unique to Chinese medicine, describes the upper burner, or chest region; the middle burner, or abdominal region; and the lower burner, or pelvic region. These burners function together as one larger, comprehensive organ to generate, warm, and distribute energy throughout the body.

Even your favorite beauty supply store couldn't arrange better door-to-door delivery of everything your body needs to keep it feeling and looking healthy, vibrant, and beautiful! This circulatory movement makes sure that each organ gets sufficient energy, essence, and blood to restore, repair, and renew itself. It also provides some guidance as to how we can rearrange our lifestyle to better fit our body's energetic rhythm.

But the meridians do more than provide a pathway for *Qi* to deliver its powerful energy boosts to specific organs. Each meridian and organ is associated with a specific set of mental, physical, and emotional functions too. Because the brain interacts with the meridians and organs in this way, the brain's health is contingent on their overall health and vice versa. Basically, the energy that is responsible for our physical health is also responsible for our mental health. The two are totally inseparable. But we'll talk more about this astounding mind-body connection in chapter 3!

YIN AND YANG

Of course, more familiar to Westerners than any of these other terms, *Yin* and *Yang* are generally understood to be the opposite yet complementary natures of energy. But their meaning is more nuanced than that. They are energies that are dependent on the other's existence for their very own existence.

For instance, *Yin* describes a cooling energy, while *Yang* describes a warming energy. We simply cannot comprehend the notion of warmth without its comparison to cold. When one is deficient, it means there is relatively too much of the other, requiring an adjustment to both. The body has its own self-regulatory system to keep *Yin* and *Yang* balanced. The classic example of this is when women hit menopause. Their Kidney *Yin* energy is significantly deficient while their *Yang* energy is in relative excess, causing them to experience hot flashes and night sweats. The same is true when exercise causes you to be too hot. In that case, your pores open to release some of that warm energy as sweat, which helps you cool down. Similarly, in the winter when your energy is excessively cold, shivering creates the internal heat necessary to warm you up.

Yin and *Yang*'s dynamic—this constant balancing act—determines our health. These two energies must be in perfect harmony for us to be completely well. Throughout this book we will show you many ways to consciously and actively achieve balanced energies, balanced health, and a balanced life.

EXTERNAL ENERGY

As I mentioned earlier, *Qi* exists outside of our bodies too, keeping the life force around us functioning optimally. There are several different types of external energies, but the predominant ones occur with the different seasons and various climates. They manifest as Wind, Dampness, Cold, Dryness, and Heat. Our body can choose how to interact with outside energies to its benefit. However, when the body's function is compromised due to internal reasons, or when the outside energy is so strong that it can break down the body's defenses, these outside forces can either cause or worsen an energetic imbalance inside the body. Essentially, when these external energies permeate the body, they have the power to change our own energetic constitution, at least for a little while. You will recall that we discussed some of these effects in chapter 1. We obviously breathe *Qi* in, but Chinese medicine explains that there are also points along the meridians that allow *Qi* to enter and exit our bodies, enhancing our communication and exchange with the world around us. These are our acupuncture points. By strategically stimulating selected points, acupuncturists can treat illness and diseases that are caused by energetic imbalances. Acupuncture and acupressure have greatly helped us refine communications between internal and external energies, and certain spa treatments are effective in doing so as well. But knowing what you wish to accomplish with these "conversations"—what you want to let in, keep out, or release from your body at all times—is incredibly important.

For instance, a forty-six-year-old patient named Judy came to me feeling as if she had aged ten years during the harsh winter. She had just moved to New Jersey from a warmer climate and was not used to the freezing temperatures and snowfall we were having. She reported feeling cold, depressed, and anxious all season. Upon talking with her further, she told me that she had stopped menstruating two years earlier, and was experiencing urinary incontinence as well. She was assessed using classical Chinese medicine techniques and was diagnosed with severe Kidney *Qi* Deficiency. Clearly, adjusting to the change in weather had exacerbated some earlier energetic imbalances and created a few new ones. The winter is particularly difficult for the Kidneys, and because they are connected to the Bladder and reproductive organs, the harsh conditions of the season can deplete their energies as well. I administered acupuncture treatments twice weekly for three months, gave her a course of Chinese herbal supplements, and changed her diet to include foods rich in nutrients known to supplement the *Qi* stored in her Kidneys. In that time her symptoms vastly improved.

Hopefully, this information helps you see that our bodies and our environment have a tremendous influence on each other and that both possess some incredibly natural and powerful tools to rejuvenate and heal us. You can also see that when the foundations of these important tools—our *Jing, Qi, and Shen*—are diminished in any way, it causes us to age. For this reason we really need to protect them and use them as equitably as we can throughout our lives. It is never too early to establish a lifestyle that encourages this behavior. The following are a few ways you can actively balance your *Qi* and support your *Jing* and *Shen*. When your vital energies are all flowing through your body as effectively as they should—moving in the right direction, sufficiently, and with balanced properties—your internal and external organs stay healthy, your emotions remain in check, your spirit radiates beauty, and nothing is demanding more of your essence for use in molecular repair than it can afford to give. You are living in a harmonious body.

EASY THINGS YOU CAN DO TO SUPPORT AND PRESERVE YOUR *JING*, *QI*, AND *SHEN*

Enjoy foods that nurture your Kidneys: In the previous chapter we suggested maintaining a balanced diet and making a concerted effort to avoid consuming the same foods (even the healthiest of choices) repeatedly. In the next chapter we'll talk specifically about the types of foods that support each organ; but for now, be sure to add some of the following foods to your diet, as they are all known to nourish your Kidneys and to replenish the *Qi* and *Jing* stored there: grains, cooked dark-green leafy vegetables, black mushrooms, black soybeans, black sesame seeds, walnuts, chestnuts, lychee nuts, seaweed, fish, shrimp, lamb, and duck are all good choices. Many herbs are also thought to support Kidney *Qi* and *Jing*. Among the most popular are ginseng and rehmannia root.

Eat when the timing is right: Your body energy is strongest at different times for different organ functions, as the chart on page 23 indicates. If you truly want to get the most nutrient value out of what you consume, schedule meals for the times when your digestion, absorption, and metabolism energies are at their peak: between 7:00 A.M. and 9:00 A.M., 11:00 A.M. and 1:00 P.M., and 5:00 P.M. and 7:00 P.M. When you eat during these times, you are allowing your body to supplement its supply of *Postnatal Jing*, easing up on your body's demands for *Prenatal Jing*. This is just one more way to help make the supply of the good stuff last longer!

By the way, one thing modern medicine and traditional Chinese medicine agree on is that skipping breakfast increases the risk of developing chronic illness, so be sure to make time for this meal! Think of eating breakfast as fortifying your *Shen* and ensuring that you have an emotionally positive start to your day too.

Cleanse your body early in the morning: Because *Qi* activity is strongest in the Large Intestine between 5:00 A.M. and 7:00 A.M., this is the best time to free your body of toxins. Before heading for the bathroom, drink a glass of warm water and massage your abdomen to help make moving your bowels easier. It is essential to good health to rid your body of waste at least once a day. Doing so when your body is most cooperative can help you meet this daily requirement.

Know when to exercise: The energies for your Kidney and Bladder Meridians are strongest between 3:00 P.M. and 7:00 P.M. These energies support agility and movement, so if you are the type of person who enjoys vigorous physical activity, this is the ideal time to exercise and still conserve energy! However, if your schedule only permits you to exercise in the morning, the body's circadian rhythms suggest that better disciplines for you might include meditation, yoga, or tai chi. A moderate level of physical exercise in the morning also helps stimulate your *Yang Qi* to rise, providing clarity of mind at the outset of the day. All three offer incredible benefits to the rest of your body as well.

Stick to an 11:00 P.M. bedtime: The hours between 11:00 P.M. and 3:00 A.M. are when your body energy nurtures your Liver and Gallbladder Meridians. These organs are major players in how well your body functions during the daytime. Allowing your body to rest and replenish throughout this period is the key to healthy living. If you are unable to keep to this schedule, note that chapter 6 extensively addresses the subject of sleep and offers many valuable suggestions as to what else you can do under these circumstances.

Keep a cool head to help balance your *Yang* energy: All *Yang Qi* meridians converge in the head to provide the brain with the energy it needs to function. But to operate on an optimal level, the brain also needs to be balanced by *Yin Qi*. Keeping your head cool really helps balance out these warming and cooling energies, and is also believed to decrease the release of detrimental neurotransmitters and other toxic substances. Brain cooling lowers the brain's need for nutrients, including oxygen and glucose. And it also appears to have therapeutic potential for treating epilepsy, stroke, asphyxia, and other neurological diseases. Lastly, it is also known to prevent brain damage after heart attacks. It seems as if keeping a cool and level head is good advice on many levels!

Warm your feet to help balance your *Yin* energy: Because your feet are far away from your Heart and your central nervous system, the blood supply to them can run thin. As a result they can become cold, constricting the energy channels that meet there. The feet are actually where *Yang* (Warm) *Qi* ends and where *Yin* (Cool) *Qi* begins. If your feet are too cold, the balance of *Yin* and *Yang* will be disturbed and your body's energy will very likely stagnate, impacting the whole body's ability to function. To keep these two energies well balanced and circulating properly, it is important to make sure your feet are kept comfortably warm, but not sweaty, as perspiration will cause valuable *Qi* to be released through your pores. Getting this just right is important for your whole body, but it is also especially helpful in preventing peripheral vascular disease and neuropathy.

Maintain a peaceful mind: Emotion is necessary for human beings to live and connect with each other. *Emotional distress,* however, depletes your body of its vital essence. It blocks and disturbs the flow of your energies, causing dysfunction on every health level—from the most internal to the most visible. Meditating can help calm and quiet the mind, ridding it of all worries, anxieties, fears, and concerns that can have a negative impact on your *Qi*.

Norma's Musings on Creative Energy

Finding out how many different kinds of internal energies there are and learning how they function opened up a whole new dimension of understanding for me. Having this kind of information seems as vital to me now as knowing your blood type, the color of your eyes, or certain genetic markers for disease. I appreciate having a greater sense of how my emotional and mental energies fuel, inspire, and affect me behaviorally. It's another layer of information that helps me define who I am.

Learning more about the concept of *Shen* was particularly interesting to me, especially its role in inspiration and creativity. We all know *creative energy* exists, but it is wonderful to encounter a medical system that formally acknowledges it. Chinese medicine understands it as more than just a figure of speech. It knows how creativity moves around within our bodies. It can track its specific pathway and influences. It confirms that creativity is born out of being connected to the larger world on many different levels. Chinese medicine has an interesting take on love and intimacy that can be applied to creative energy too. It teaches us that when you engage with someone you care for deeply, the exchange multiplies your energies. Similarly, when you do something you love creatively and share that experience or its results with others, it seems to generate energy, not just within yourself, but in the people around you as well. It's contagious energy. Of course, the reverse is true too. When you do something you don't like, such as taking part in a project just for the money, the burnout rate is rapid. The effort saps your energy, and others perceive that drain in your actions and appearance. It seems like an ever-important reminder to do what you love. Using your creative energy wisely is good for your own life-sustaining energies and for those of the people around you as well.

For me, this closer look at our internal energies also emphasizes how much we can do physically to supplement them. I happen to exercise every day at exactly the time Dr. Yang says it is optimal to, and I've found it's really good for me. I also love to sleep and always feel inspired after a good night's rest. The fact that energy is being delivered to organs that enhance specific functions at precise times while I'm sleeping explains this phenomenon. It should also make everyone want to go to sleep within the time frame Dr. Yang suggests. In fact, one of the most amazing benefits of the acupuncture treatment I received from Dr. Yang was the quality of rest I had as a result. Acupuncture, just like sleep, is all about sending healing energies to the organs and systems that need them most. During my sessions I had some of the best sleep of my life. If only Michael Jackson had known about these profound effects! If you have a fear of needles, the one thing that might entice you to try acupuncture is the amazing, revitalizing slumber it induces and how completely rested and restored you look afterward. I must tell you that the needles are so fine I barely ever feel a pinprick as they go in—and if I do, my body acclimates quickly because it understands that the point being worked on is connected to a part of me that needs some extra care and attention. In that case I might think, *Whoa, that one was tricky*, but then I usually feel my body giving in to the sensation because it knows the feeling is promoting healing. In a matter of minutes I'm drifting off and then it's as if I'm under anesthesia. How could you possibly sleep like that if the process hurts? If you still have doubts, consider the fact that wearing a pair of gorgeous Jimmy Choos or Louboutins for a night out dancing is far more painful, and we seem to have no problem with that!

3

Organ-ization

Now that our readers are over the initial shock of learning that there is a formal energetic dimension to our bodies that even most of our doctors missed studying, they're probably asking themselves, *What else didn't I learn in seventh-grade biology?* You hint in the previous chapter that classical Chinese medicine views our organ functions differently too. **Could you please explain those differences and what impact they have on our total health and beauty?**

Absolutely. Classical Chinese medicine is full of surprises, as you say. And one of the biggest surprises—even to some of your favorite science teachers—involves the organs.

As I mentioned earlier, the meridians carry physical, mental, emotional, and spiritual energies to and from the various organs. From that bit of information alone, one can tell that the organs fulfill a three-times greater role than modern medicine ascribes to them.

To make this crystal clear, let's break those roles down for you. Admittedly, this is a lot of new information to digest, so I ask that you follow along with me step by step through this chapter and the next. I promise all the pieces will come together in a classical chart found on pages 72 to 73 that neatly summarizes and illustrates how energy works within us . . . and in exchange with the wider universe too.

THE ORGANS' PHYSICAL ROLES

Chinese medicine identifies five organs—the Liver, Heart, Spleen, Lungs, and Kidneys—as our *primary organs*. Each of them works in tandem with a *partner organ*.

The Liver's partner organ is the Gallbladder.
The Heart's partner organ is the Small Intestine.
The Spleen's partner organ is the Stomach.
The Lungs' partner organ is the Large Intestine.
The Kidneys' partner organ is the Urinary Bladder.

These pairings have a *Yin-and-Yang* relationship in that they fulfill complementary functions. The primary organs transform, regulate, and store *Jing, Qi*, blood, and body fluids, whereas the partner organs digest, stimulate, and transport them. Primary organs tend to be solid, while partner organs are generally hollow. It is essential for the maintenance of good health that the functions of each organ in a pairing remain balanced.

Primary and Partner Organs at a Glance

PRIMARY ORGAN	STATE	PARTNER ORGAN	STATE
Liver	*Yin*/Solid Organ	Gallbladder	*Yang*/Hollow Organ
Heart	*Yin*/Solid Organ	Small Intestine	*Yang*/Hollow Organ

PRIMARY ORGAN	STATE	PARTNER ORGAN	STATE
Spleen	*Yin*/Solid Organ	Stomach	*Yang*/Hollow Organ
Lungs	*Yin*/Solid Organ	Large Intestine	*Yang*/Hollow Organ
Kidneys	*Yin*/Solid Organ	Urinary Bladder	*Yang*/Hollow Organ

Now here's where you can finally begin to see the association between our internal health and our exterior beauty, among other amazing connections.

According to modern medicine, the Liver's main function is to biochemically metabolize and detoxify food and medications, but Chinese medicine believes that, in conjunction with the Gallbladder, it also energetically directs the flow of *Qi* throughout the body. Additionally, it is in charge of your eyes and vision, your tendons and ligaments, as well as your nails. It also regulates your tears, digestion, sleep, and menstruation if you are a woman. That's right—in addition to having a good night's sleep, getting the most nutrients out of what you eat, and having more regular and less painful periods—**keeping your Liver and Gallbladder healthy can mean having vibrant eyes, strong fingernails, and the kind of healthy connective tissue that ensures naturally firm and elastic skin too.**

Similarly, in modern medicine, the Heart's main function is to biochemically pump blood through the circulatory system so it can be oxygenated in the Lungs, but Chinese medicine believes that, in conjunction with your Small Intestine, it also energetically oversees your nervous system; it governs your tongue and speech; it fortifies your veins and arteries; and it regulates your sweat and enhances your complexion. **Yes, keeping your Heart and Small Intestine healthy can help restore color to your cheeks. It can even give you that fresh-faced look you prized so much in your youth.**

As for the Spleen, modern medicine believes its main function is to biochemically purify your blood and help your immune system identify and attack foreign antigens and disease, but Chinese medicine believes that, in conjunction with the Stomach, it also energetically oversees digestion, absorption, and metabolism; regulates your saliva; keeps your taste buds sharp and your mouth healthy and free of germs; and fortifies your muscles, flesh, and lips. **In terms of beauty, a healthy Spleen and Stomach can help you maintain shapely arms and legs as well as a kissable smile.**

Similarly, in modern medicine, the Lungs' main function is to biochemically provide you with energy in the form of oxygen and cleanse your body of waste in the form of carbon dioxide, but Chinese medicine believes that, in conjunction with the Large Intestine, they also energetically regulate mucus and water retention throughout your body, keep your nose clear and healthy, maintain your sense of smell, and fortify your skin and body hair. **In many ways, taking care of your Lungs and Large Intestine can keep you wrinkle and dry-patch free.**

Lastly, in modern medicine, the Kidneys' main function is to biochemically filter waste and excess water from your blood, but Chinese medicine believes that, in conjunction with the Urinary Bladder, they also energetically direct your development, fertility, reproduction, and sexual functions; they make sure your ears are healthy and that your hearing is impeccable; and they fortify your bones and head hair. **When your Kidneys and Bladder remain healthy, you will enjoy a lustrous mane, you will delay the graying of your hair, and you will have fuller eyelashes and brows for a lot longer than you might have expected.**

Organ and Beauty Correlations at a Glance

PRIMARY ORGAN	Liver	Heart	Spleen	Lungs	Kidneys
PARTNER ORGAN	Gallbladder	Small Intestine	Stomach	Large Intestine	Urinary Bladder

SENSORY ORGAN AND SENSE	Eyes Vision	Tongue Speech	Mouth Taste	Nose Smell	Ears Hearing
RELATED ORGANS	Tendons, Ligaments	Pulse, Veins, Arteries	Muscles, Flesh	Skin	Bones, Joints
EXTERNAL MANIFESTATION	Nails	Complexion	Lips	Body Hair	Head Hair

THE ORGANS' MENTAL AND SPIRITUAL ROLES

Chinese medicine also teaches us that the five major internal organs are not only where *Qi* and *Jing* are stored, but are also the residence for human spiritual and mental functions. The Heart is very much like an emperor. It houses the *Shen,* which is the center for perception, cognition, emotion, language, and consciousness. It makes the decisions that respond to our realities, and ultimately determines our behavior. The other four organs play supportive roles for the Heart, helping to fulfill its goals and unconsciously influencing its decisions and resulting actions. **When you have a healthy Heart, you will also have spirited eyes, an assertive and joyful demeanor, a clear sense of meaning and purpose in your life, and an ability to articulate your desires. You will be full of passion in all that you do, which will provide you with the amazing power of attraction!**

The Lungs fill the role of prime minister. They house the *Po* (魄)—the corporal soul governing the body or the part of *Shen* that informs our sensory and motor functions as well as our build and physical demeanor. *Po* also encourages mental discipline, order and sensitivity, and depends not only on the *Qi* but also on the *Jing* to function. **When you take good care of your Lungs, you will have a strong sense of reality; you will be reliable and dependable in interpersonal relationships; you will build and maintain a healthy body as well as an optimistic and positive attitude. People will love to be around you!**

The Liver is most like a general. It houses the *Hun* (魂)—the ethereal soul, which, in contrast to *Po*, manifests independently of the body. It is the part of *Shen* that is able to travel beyond matter, time, and dimension. Because it is not limited by our physical sensory faculties, it enables us to reach a higher consciousness. It provides vision, strategy, and tactics to our mental functioning so we can achieve the goals that are most cherished by our Heart. *Hun* appears in our life as dreams, intuition, and inspiration. **When your Liver is healthy, you will be relaxed, wise, creative, and compassionate. You will love to share your wisdom with other people and they will not only listen, they will perceive you as a visionary!**

The Spleen is most like a minister overseeing the storage and distribution of nutritional supplies to the entire body. It also houses *Yi* (意), which includes our thoughts, ideas, and intentions. The Spleen further processes these thoughts and formulates them into a feasible plan, of course, with the help of the Liver. **When you have a healthy Spleen, you will live in the here and now; you will enjoy nurturing yourself and others with healthy gourmet foods; and you will have a clear sense of direction in life. People will find that they need you and that your happiness is contagious!**

The Kidneys house *Prenatal Jing* and *Qi* as well as *Zhi* (志). *Zhi* is the part of *Shen* that provides the determination and willpower to execute the ideas and plan that *Yi* produces. As you can see, the Kidneys contribute a great deal to our ultimate success in life. **When your Kidneys are healthy, you will radiate strength, determination, deep motivation, and dignity in all of life's endeavors. People will admire and rely on you for your leadership skills.**

So right about now, I'm sure you're wondering, *If each of these organs assume the responsibilities Western medicine collectively ascribes to the brain, what is the brain's role in Chinese medicine? Is it important at all? Or is it simply forgotten?*

You are right to ask these questions, but let me assure you that the brain is extremely important in *all* the spiritual and mental functions of the body. It is known as the sea of the marrow, and is one of the most special organs we have. However, its function depends on the energetic connections it maintains with each of the internal organs that are part of the body's energetic network. Different organ systems connect with different parts of the brain and are responsible for specific functions of the brain. **So take good care of your internal organs, and your brain will take care of itself!**

Organ and Mental and Spiritual Correlations at a Glance

PRIMARY ORGAN	Liver	Heart	Spleen	Lungs	Kidneys
PARTNER ORGAN	Gallbladder	Small Intestine	Stomach	Large Intestine	Urinary Bladder
SPIRITUAL AND MENTAL FUNCTIONS	*Hun* (The Ethereal Soul) Vision, Decision Making, Strategy, Judgment	*Shen* (The Emperor of the Soul) Consciousness, Perception, Cognition, Emotion, Language, Initiative	*Yi* (The Mindful Soul) Thoughts, Ideas, Intention, Reasoning	*Po* (The Corporal Soul) Mental Discipline, Order, Sensitivity, Restraint	*Zhi* (The Willful Soul) Motivation, Determination, Willpower, Coordination
MENTAL QUALITY	Sensitivity	Creativity	Clarity	Intuition	Spontaneity

THE ORGANS' EMOTIONAL ROLES

This is usually the part where people have a big *aha* moment. Emotion is a very strong energetic experience. It packs a lot of power. While modern medicine generally acknowledges emotion's impact on the body, Chinese medicine teaches us that each primary organ is associated with a specific emotion.

The Liver is associated with anger.

The Heart is associated with joy.

The Spleen is associated with worry.

The Lungs are associated with grief.

The Kidneys are associated with fear.

This means that when an emotion becomes excessive or out of control, it can disturb the energy flowing to the organ associated with it and negatively impact our mind, body, and spirit. For instance, excessive anger or resentment will actually damage your Liver and its partner organ, the Gallbladder. Sadness and grief can have a tremendous impact on your Lungs and their partner organ, the Large Intestine. Worry will deliver a one-two punch to the Spleen and its partner organ, the Stomach. (Ever wonder why stress leads to ulcers?!) Fear will consume the energy of your Kidneys and Bladder. And even excessive joy—presenting as overexcitement or mania—can harm the Heart and Small Intestine.

This powerful impact works the other way around too: if your system is compromised due to a bad lifestyle, poor diet, physical trauma, or infection, then you will be emotionally compromised as well, meaning that you will tend to experience more of these difficult emotions than usual.

What happened to a thirty-six-year-old patient named Paul is a great example of how physical states really impact emotional states and vice versa.

PATIENT-TESTED TRUTHS

Paul had tried everything to help alleviate sciatic pain radiating down to his right leg and ankle along his Gallbladder Meridian. His doctor recommended that he undergo surgery to remove the herniated disc in his lower back that might have been causing the pain. Despite battling these flare-ups for years, he desperately wanted to find a different solution. "Going under the knife" terrified him. After Paul was treated with natural herbal supplements and several courses of acupuncture, the pain completely disappeared. In the process, Paul and his wife noticed a marked difference in his mood too. Paul had always been a bitter guy who harbored a lot of anger and resentment. The smallest offense would set him off. After the treatments, he became a much more tolerant man. His colleagues and his boss couldn't believe how much he had mellowed. Paul even buried the hatchet with family members over a long-standing disagreement he had with them.

Another equally powerful example comes from a twenty-two-year-old patient named Suzie who heard that acupuncture could help ease her anxiety. She suffered from bouts of it all throughout college and was now headed to law school. She wanted to find a way to curb or control her fears once and for all. After several treatments she not only felt more relaxed, she reported that her chronic urinary tract infections had ceased too!

Organ and Emotion Correlations at a Glance

PRIMARY ORGAN	Liver	Heart	Spleen	Lungs	Kidneys
PARTNER ORGAN	Gallbladder	Small Intestine	Stomach	Large Intestine	Urinary Bladder
EMOTION	Anger	Joy	Worry	Grief	Fear

EASY THINGS YOU CAN DO TO NURTURE EACH OF YOUR PRIMARY ORGANS RIGHT AWAY!

To support your Liver:

Avoid interactions with people who are ill tempered and who frustrate or irritate you.

Their energies tend to block yours!

Practice tolerance with others and go easy on yourself as well. Judgment's negativity lodges in your Liver where it can be incredibly damaging. Self-effacing thoughts and comments can wreck havoc too.

Reduce the intake of alcohol and coffee. Small amounts of alcohol often help to circulate *Qi* and blood, and are sometimes used as an initial facilitator for Chinese herbal remedies. However, repetitive alcohol consumption, especially in large quantities, generates Heat and Dampness in your body, and stresses your Liver energy. Consequently, it can muddle your Heart energy and disturb your *Shen*. Similarly, too much coffee puts stress on your Liver and tightens the muscles of your neck and shoulders. Although people enjoy drinking it because it stimulates mind energy, too much coffee can increase the perception of emotional stress and reactivity and can keep people awake at night during the very time that the Liver and Gallbladder need to rest the most. Enjoy it, but do so in moderation and during the earlier hours of the day.

Add leafy green vegetables to your diet. Kale, spinach, collard greens, watercress, and chard are a few good choices. All vegetables harness energy from the sun, but your Liver *Qi* really prizes leafy green varieties. As you will discover in later sections, the Liver's energy responds especially well to the color cyan (a mix of green and blue) and to the spring season in general.

Be sure to get your best sleep between the hours of 11:00 P.M. and 3:00 A.M. Again, this is when your *Qi* is doing its nightly repair work on your Liver.

Massage your Liver 3 acupuncture point. It will help keep your Liver *Qi* flowing smoothly and in the right direction. Find the point (see illustration on page 43) on the dorsum of the foot in a depression distal to the junctions of the first and second metatarsal bones. (Don't let these terms confuse you. The picture I've provided is really all the help you'll need to find the exact location, but I always prefer to be precise! I never know when I could be inspiring a future acupuncturist.) Next, apply firm pressure while massaging the point for five minutes. Press when you breathe in and release when you breathe out. Do this two times a day. You should feel a dull ache, soreness and even numbness as you press on the point. That lets you know that you are on the right spot and that you are actively stimulating *Qi*'s movement along the Liver Meridian.

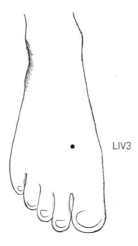

LIV3

Drink my "Love Your Liver" tea. Place 12 goji berries, 6 dried chrysanthemums, 3 dried roses, and 3 grams of green tea (preferably decaffeinated) in a teapot with 6½ cups of hot water and simmer for 5 minutes. Sipping this tea will soothe and replenish your Liver *Qi.*

To support your Heart:

Maintain a joyful spirit without becoming overly excited. Surrounding yourself with those who make you feel good, engaging in activities that help others, and remembering to show gratitude for the people and experiences that enhance your life are just a few ways you can do this.

Practice wisdom and truthfulness. Nothing burdens the Heart more than saying or doing something you are uncomfortable with on a deeper level. Being honest is the best way to be Heart smart.

Moderate your intake of hot and spicy foods. These foods generally add warming energy to the Heart and uplift people's spirit. However, if eaten in excess, they can generate too much Heat, turbo-charging your *Shen,* kindling fiery emotions, and leading to anxiety, insomnia, and even palpitations.

Increase bitter and red-colored vegetables in your diet. Bitterness is an energy of taste that nurtures the Heart, and the same is true of the color red. Foods such as chard, endive, watercress, artichokes, asparagus, rhubarb, lemons, grapefruit, beets, tomatoes, radishes, and red peppers help reduce Heat and calm the Heart. Nature makes it easy for you to remember some of these foods by coordinating their color to the one most associated with the Heart!

Set aside some time between 11:00 A.M. and 1:00 P.M. to relax. Taking a nap or meditating during this window of time is ideal because this is when your *Qi* is most actively attending to your Heart.

Massage your Heart 7 acupuncture point. This will clear the way for your Heart *Qi* to do what it does best. Find the point (see illustration below) at the first wrist crease, on the radial side of the flexor carpi ulnaris tendon, between the ulna and the pisiform bones. (Your friends and family will be wildly impressed that you know this jargon when you demonstrate for them how to be Heart healthy too!) Again, apply firm pressure when massaging this point for five minutes two times a day. If you have done it right, you will feel a dull ache, soreness, and some numbness there. Massaging this point activates the *Qi* to flow more freely along the Heart Meridian.

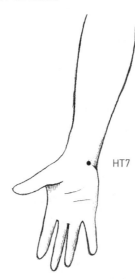

HT7

Drink my "Love Your Heart" tea. Add 6 grams of bulbus lilii, 5 red dates, 10 grams of arillus longan, 6 grams of American ginseng, and 3 grams of green tea (preferably decaffeinated) to 6½ cups of water and simmer for ten minutes. This tea will warm your Heart, nurture its *Qi* and blood, and relax and pacify your mind. Some of the harder-to-find ingredients can be purchased online.

To support your Spleen:

Watch out for "what if" thoughts. Focusing on the things you have control over in the here and now will help you break the worry habit that is so damaging to the Spleen.

Practice compassion for yourself as well as others. Just as a healthy Spleen provides you with clarity, reason, and purpose, exercising those important qualities reinvigorates your Spleen's health and energies too. Remember that healing works both ways!

Reduce fatty foods and those containing refined sugars. The Spleen and its partner organ, the Stomach, serve as a "cooker" for the body, allowing it to readily absorb nutrients from the foods you eat. These organs need Warm and Damp energy to break down food. However, excessive Dampness, due to the overconsumption of fatty, greasy, oily, and sugary foods, prevents the Spleen from extracting the necessary essence and *Qi* from our food. Minimizing these foods will help these organs function far better.

Increase warm foods and yellow-colored vegetables in your diet. The energy of the color yellow nurtures the Spleen. Enjoy eating grapefruit, cooked summer squash, butternut squash, peppers, yams, and carrots, as they all help to warm Spleen *Qi* and break down any thick fluids impeding its movement.

Be mindful and productive between the hours of 9:00 A.M. and 11:00 A.M. This is when *Qi* is most actively attending to the Spleen, so your mental acuity is apt to be at its highest. Make the most of the opportunity by scheduling concentrated tasks at this time.

Massage your Spleen 3 acupuncture point. This will help your Spleen *Qi* get out of any sticky situations that may arise! That point (see illustration below) is located at the medial aspect of the foot, in the depression posterior and inferior to the proximal metatarso-digital joint of the big toe, at the junction of the lighter and darker skin. Yes, right there. As always, apply firm pressure, massaging the point with your thumb for five minutes, two times a day.

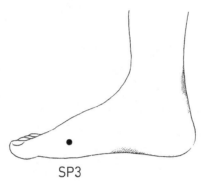

SP3

Drink my "Love Your Spleen" tea. Place 10 grams of *dang shen*, 10 grams of *bai zhu*, 10 grams of *maiya*, and 10 grams of *chenpi* with or without black tea and 6½ cups of water in a teapot and heat for ten minutes. Drink this tea throughout the day. It will energize your Spleen *Qi*, increase your digestion and metabolism, and reduce Dampness and water retention in your body. And yes, it will also help you lose weight!

To support your Lungs:

Manage feelings of loss, grief, and sadness. While you need to give yourself time to literally catch your breath after a traumatic life event, it is important not to become debilitated by the event. Prolonged sorrow can weigh heavily on your Lungs and compromise your immune system, causing all kinds of upper respiratory problems.

Practice letting go and being open minded. In the same way that lifting a heavy weight can leave you short of breath, carrying a heavy emotional burden can have a similar effect. You must free yourself of that burden and be optimistic that, in time, something positive will come and help fill the void.

Make a conscious effort to breathe in fresh air. All too many of us get so busy we tend to forget to breathe deeply throughout the day and even while taking walks. We also forget to engage in more exercises that utilize cleansing breaths; to water the plants that oxygenate our homes; to keep our living and work spaces free of dust, fumes, germs, and other irritants; and to use a humidifier when the air around us is too Dry or a dehumidifier when it is too Damp. However, these are important things to remember. We all have to actively do our part to increase the quality of the air around us.

Add more white-colored vegetables to your diet. White light is the airiest of energies. It is infused in mushrooms, leeks, onions, garlic, fennel, turnips, parsnips, and endive, all of which enhance your Lung *Qi* and help you breathe easier. Allergy sufferers and those who get frequent colds may want to add some of these to their diet at the first signs of trouble, or as a preventative measure.

Stay warm at night and do not set your alarm for earlier than 5:00 in the morning. *Qi* revitalizes the Lungs between the hours of 3:00 A.M. and 5:00 A.M. each day. Having restful and warm sleep at that time will help "clear the air," at least internally.

Massage your Lung 9 acupuncture point. This will help your Lung *Qi* breeze through your system smoothly. You can find this point (see illustration on page 48) on the radial end of the transverse crease of the wrist, where the radial artery pulsates. Apply firm pressure to the level of your tolerance as a dull ache sets in, then massage the point for five minutes, two times a day.

Drink my "Love Your Lungs" tea. Place 10 grams of *sha shen,* 10 grams of *huang qi,* 10 grams of *mai dong,* and 10 grams of *xing ren* with or without 3 grams of green tea in a teapot with 6½ cups of water, then heat for ten minutes. This will yield a one-day supply. This tea is known to improve your immunity, to reduce allergies, and generally to help you breathe deeper and more effectively.

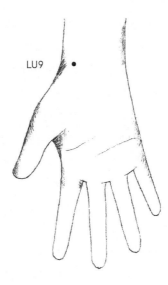

LU9

To support your Kidneys:

Manage your fears. Anxieties related to work, school, personal relationships, finances, emotional trauma, the death of a loved one, or a serious medical illness can all put unrelenting strain on your Kidneys. Given what an important role your Kidneys play in your present vigor and in your longevity, as well as in the health of your future children, it is important to learn to release your fears. One of the best things you can do, besides breathing deeply, is to engage in an activity that changes the channel in your mind, taking the attention off the issue you are ruminating about. Watch a movie—comedies and mysteries are especially distracting. If there is a solution to the problem you are focused on, work your way through it step-by-step, proving to yourself that fears can be faced and overcome.

Stay motivated and remember to practice courage and willpower. As the keeper of our life force, the Kidneys are concerned with the quality of our life now *and* in the future. These three attributes—motivation, ambition, and willpower—move us closer to fulfillment of that vitality.

Add more black-colored fruits and vegetables to your diet. While I suggested a variety of different foods to support your *Qi* in chapter 2, there are lots of other options to help boost your Kidney *Qi* and *Jing*. Blackberries, black figs, dark cherries, dark grapes, plums, prunes, raisins, and vanilla beans are also delicious and healthful.

Drink a sufficient amount of water and control the amount of salty foods you consume. Now that I've made several suggestions as to what you can *eat* to nourish your Kidneys I should really tell you what to *drink*. Since the Kidneys are a cooling organ, water is vital to helping them reduce excessive Heat throughout the body. Menopausal women: you should heed this advice more than most. As you age and deplete your *Prenatal Jing* supply, you can become Kidney *Yin* deficient, causing your reproductive organs to overheat. This is essentially what your hot flashes are all about. Drinking water and regulating your salt intake can help.

Enjoy a healthy, balanced sex life. Sex invigorates the *Qi* and keeps it circulating, but since the *Prenatal Jing* stored in the Kidneys is intended to aid in reproduction, every time men ejaculate, they are giving away some of their life-force energy—the *Prenatal Jing* intended for the vitality of their offspring and for their own sustained vitality later in life. Excessive sex will deplete those stores of *Jing* at a more rapid pace. Of course, what constitutes excess is different for every person. If you find that you are lethargic, you have absolutely no energy, or that you are unable to concentrate the day after, then you have engaged in too much. You might consider withholding ejaculation during intercourse from time to time. Seminal retention can help reserve some of that potentially lost *Jing* and even heighten the sexual experience.

Adolescent boys who masturbate a great deal will often find that their school grades are slipping because they have also released significant reserves of their life-force energy that are essential for maintaining good concentration and memory. They needn't stop all together, but they should reduce the frequency of their masturbation or masturbate up to the point of orgasm or ejaculation.

On a related note, every month when women menstruate they give away some of the *Prenatal Jing* intended for the life that the ovum they are now passing would have carried had it been impregnated. If your blood flow is particularly heavy at this time, you may want to seek help from a Chinese medicine practitioner or an acupuncturist who can help guide the further nourishment of your Kidneys. This is especially true if your period brings on greater depression, anxiety, or moodiness than it does for others. It may be that your Kidney *Qi* is deficient and that you are losing too much of your vital essence at this time.

Massage your Kidney 3 acupuncture point. The prospect of a long life resides in your Kidneys, and with the help of acupressure, it's at your fingertips too. The point you are looking for (see illustration below) is located in the depression midway between the tip of the medial malleolus and the attachment of the Achilles tendon. Massage it the same way you were instructed to do with all the other points already listed—for five minutes, two times a day.

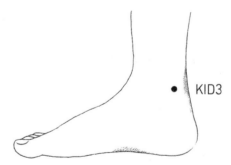

Drink my "Love Your Kidneys" tea. Place 10 grams of *ren shen*, 10 grams of *he tao ren*, 10 grams of *du zhong ye*, 10 grams of *shan yu rou*, 10 grams of *wu wei zi* in a teapot with 6½ cups of water and heat for ten minutes. This tea will restore your energy and motivation, reduce your lower back pain and anxiety, and enhance your libido and sexual sensation.

Norma's Musings on How to Deal with Fear, Anger, and Worry

Of all the advice we're ever offered, being told to rid ourselves of negative energy and to minimize emotional stress are probably the two suggestions that can make the greatest difference. Doctors tell us this all the time, but it seems even more relevant when you can identify the vital organs that each emotion affects, as Chinese medicine does. Of course, accomplishing this task is always easier said than done. Some of the biggest obstacles that I find people encounter are fear and anger. To combat these, there are a few things I do that might help you too.

I genuinely try to never let fear stop me from doing something I want to do. I accept that half of my day will be spent preventing problems while the other half will be spent solving them, so I'm never really shocked if something goes wrong. To minimize that possibility, I am always thinking ahead as much as I can. That helps me anticipate and avert problems before they ever happen. I tell myself, *The better I get at preventing problems, the more time I'll have to explore new opportunities.* When you get better at preventing problems, you also get better at finding solutions to the ones that slip through. And sometimes these solutions are more creative and effective than anything you would have come up with if the problem never arose. So, for me, having a problem can sometimes be a good thing—a reason to innovate. You have to operate this way in the fashion industry— and many other industries—or you just die.

When I see people neglecting to do the things they want to do because they have too much fear of things going wrong and failing—they never have the gratifying experiences they should, and they never reach their full potential either. Anyone who has ever done anything with a degree of success will tell you it's the problems and negative experiences that helped them get smarter, evolve, and ultimately become better at what they do. So for the sake of living more fully and looking more enlivened because you are indeed living, embrace your dreams. Recognize that things will go wrong; then put your mind at ease by developing contingency plans for when they do. Prepare yourself to say, "Hmm, how am I going to creatively get around this now?" And also be prepared to have a better idea than you ever thought you could have. This is a way I like to deal with fear. Resist the impulse to shut down your brain and body. That will only isolate you, rob you of some amazing life adventures, and prevent you from having the unlimited creative experiences you deserve.

Because fear and anger are two horrible states that go hand in hand, when you deal with your fear problem, you will also deal with your anger problem. Anger usually results from being too afraid to do something of importance to you. It is rarely because an effort went wrong. More often than not, it's because you never dared to dream the big dream—preventing an extraordinary opportunity to do things that can change your life. I think many people get frustrated with themselves for not feeling worthy of big dreams and actually blame other people. Often they become angry and unhappy. It is possible to create illness physically and emotionally when we hold on to anger.

Worry is also linked to fear. But in my opinion, a little worry is okay. Not too much, of course—it's all in how you use it that matters. Worry is there to let you know you need a plan and a strong backup solution. In the correct measure, it's a catalyst for getting things done right. The best way to curb worry is to act on it and review your work until it meets your standards, then let it go. The good kind of worry helps athletes; it helps performers; it helps geniuses. For me there is also a real synergy between worry and anticipation. If I am worried about something but don't address it right away, I have to go back to make it better before I can move on. I usually approach my dreams or ideas concerned that someone else won't like them. But if I believe in my idea, I should be able to sell the concept. If there is resistance to the idea, I try to study it and understand the reason for it. I don't ignore feedback. I incorporate it without changing the integrity of my idea. Then worry evolves into anticipation. It's that wonderful space where meeting a challenge melds into waiting for the positive results. I can assure you that getting a grip on fear builds confidence. The power of confidence is that you stand straighter, smile more, and breathe better! Away go the frown lines. You become a more loving person and interact with others in a more relaxed way.

4

Health, Beauty, and Wellness by the Numbers

USING THE POWER OF FIVE TO NATURALLY ENHANCE YOUR VITALITY, SPIRIT, AND APPEARANCE

Dr. Yang, now that we all have a better grasp on our internal energy, what should we **know about our** interactions with the *external* world? Are there any other factors within the natural universe besides Heat, Cold, Dampness, Dryness, and Wind that we should be aware of? Are there any other elements we should invite into our bodies more frequently to prevent our aging or to promote our healing?

To provide a meaningful answer to Norma's questions, I have to ask you to participate in a brief exercise. Please put this book down for a few minutes and just observe the world around you. To help you focus, look only for the various groupings of five that exist naturally in the universe. I assure you the group including Heat, Cold, Dampness, Dryness, and Wind is just one of many examples.

Now that you are back from your momentary expedition, did you happen to list the five elements? The five senses? The five primary colors? The five primary tastes? The five primary smells? The five primary musical notes? Or the five seasons? (Of course, if you thought there were only four seasons, you must remember that Chinese medicine sees more of the world than everyone else! But we'll talk more about that later.)

THE FIVE ELEMENTS

When the originators of traditional Chinese medicine first surveyed nature, they noticed all of these groupings, and many others as well. Groups of five seem to abound in the natural world. It's quite a phenomenon. However, the group that stirred their curiosity the most was a set of elements including Wood, Fire, Earth, Metal, and Water.

What drew the attention of the originators of traditional Chinese medicine to these particular elements was their visible relationship to each other. They noticed that these elements exerted certain controlling and generating influences upon each other. When Water provides nourishment for trees, it generates Wood; when Wood is used as kindling, it generates Fire; when Fire turns to ashes, it generates Earth; when Earth's minerals are mined, they generate Metals; when Metals are melted, they generate liquid. Conversely, in the controlling cycle, Fire melts Metal; Metal cuts Wood; Wood—in the form of a tree's roots—pierces Earth; Earth dams the flow of Water; and Water extinguishes Fire.

The human body and the natural elements all operate in accordance with this generating and controlling principle for the sake of maintaining balance and ensuring that the motion of energy never ceases.

To see how this works, we simply have to look more closely at the relationship between some of the above-mentioned groups of five and our primary organs.

Chinese medicine teaches us that each of these elements can be used to help preserve, heal, and nourish the human organ most like it in character and purpose.

Wood, for instance, is associated with the Liver. Trees grow and expand upward in the same way that the Liver's *Qi* rises within the body. Trees don't like anything to block their development. They require lots of nourishment and are very sensitive to any adversarial energy that could impede their growth and function. They are also responsible for cleansing and detoxifying their environment, and when they become kindling, they are a source of warming energy. The parallels between what Wood does for nature and what the Liver does for the body are quite strong.

Fire is associated with the Heart. Their common functionality is also clear—Fire generates Heat, just as the Heart warms the entire body via blood circulation. Fire also manifests as passion and excitement that is deeply rooted in one's Heart.

Earth is associated with the Spleen. Just as everything nourishing grows from the earth, everything of nutrient value is provided to the rest of the body by the Spleen and its partner organ, the Stomach.

Metal is associated with the Lungs. The two share a remarkably similar nature in that they must both be kept clean and in fine condition to perform their jobs well.

Water is associated with the Kidneys. Here, too, the similarities are quite evident. The Kidneys function like a humidifier through which the body's water flows, is filtered to remove toxins, and is converted into a form that can readily move throughout the body the way mist permeates the air.

Organ and Element Correlations at a Glance

PRIMARY ORGAN	Liver	Heart	Spleen	Lungs	Kidneys
PARTNER ORGAN	Gallbladder	Small Intestine	Stomach	Large Intestine	Urinary Bladder
ELEMENT	Wood	Fire	Earth	Metal	Water

EASY THINGS YOU CAN DO USING THESE ELEMENTS TO NURTURE YOUR ORGANS

Wear a piece of wooden jewelry. This is especially helpful in the **springtime**—the season known for the rebirth of all nature. Earrings, necklaces, or bangle bracelets made from natural and polished woods not only make bold fashion statements, they also generate energy that does wonders for your Liver! As an added bonus, Wood can relieve you of any negative energy you may be feeling, such as irritation, anger, or rage.

Dress in breathable fabrics. To maintain Heart health you will want to fan or flame the internal fires according to the season. Wearing lighter cottons, linens, and airy blends in the **summer** allows the pores of your skin to remain open to the environment, releasing perspiration and keeping your Heart from overheating; whereas dressing in heavy layers during the winter months traps a coat of air around your body, warming and insulating it just enough to help your Heart maintain its *Yang* (Warm) energy. Successfully fanning or flaming the energy of the Heart will prevent mood swings and help you achieve a more balanced sense of joy and wonderment.

Take a mud bath. This earthly delight will pamper your Spleen, especially in the **late summer.** If a spa near you doesn't offer this option, shop for a facial mud mask at your local health store instead. I have seen some brands on the market that are made from a mix of golden root and the soft clay of China, which are both known to ease your cares and worries. Feel free to take up pottery as a hobby or to get your fingers dirty in the garden for the same effects.

Add jewelry made of precious metals to your accessories wardrobe. This is especially true in the **fall** weather. The energies of precious metals will help clear your Lungs and moisten your dry nose and throat. They also help *cut you free* from the burdensome feelings of loss and sadness. But be sure to stick to the highest quality metals, such as 18-karat gold, sterling silver, and titanium—and avoid costume jewelry as it all too often contains toxic metals.

Soak in a warm tub. Luxuriating in a long, hot bath—especially in the **winter**—is no longer a guilty pleasure. Instead, view it as a very necessary way to nurture your Kidneys. It literally washes away fears and anxieties. Indoor swimming, visiting hot springs, and spending time in a steam sauna can help too.

THE FIVE PRIMARY COLORS

Chinese medicine also teaches that various colors reflect the energies of light that correlate with a different human organ, supporting that organ's function. This is why in earlier chapters I suggested that you eat certain colored foods to aid and support different organs. We tend to think of eating as mostly a taste experience, but remember food is intended to fuel our bodies—to provide them with energy. Color delivers some of that energy through food, and as you will see, through other matter as well. The following colors are paired with the following organs:

Cyan (a mix of green and blue) correlates with the Liver. These are the colors of leaves that sprout from the wood of a wide range of trees from oak to spruce. The energy of these colors nourishes the Liver just as the energy of Wood does.

Red correlates with the Heart. Red is the color of Fire. The energy of this color warms and nourishes the Heart, which in turn warms and nourishes the entire body, just as the energy of Fire does.

Yellow correlates with the Spleen. Yellow is the color of the Earth when it lies fallow, its straw ground cover cultivating healthy soil for a future harvest. The energy of this color nourishes the Spleen, just as the energy of Earth does.

White correlates with the Lungs. White is the color of shining Metal when it is pure and well polished. The energy of this color nourishes the Lungs just as the energy of Metal does.

Black correlates with the Kidneys. Black is the absorption of all colors' energies and the color of the deepest waters. It is incredibly potent and therefore considered the color of our life force. The energy of this color nourishes the Kidneys just as the energy of Water does.

EASY THINGS YOU CAN DO USING THESE COLORS TO NURTURE YOUR ORGANS

Add color to your wardrobe as follows:

Wearing cyan-colored clothing and accessories is a wonderful way to soothe your Liver. This is especially true in the **spring** when your Liver needs more sustenance to regenerate and repair from the harsh effects of winter. Cyan's energy, just like the energy of Wood, can also help rid you of destructive emotions, such as anger or resentment, which you may have stored away during the preceding winter when you couldn't get outside to exercise more and release them. When you use this exhilarating color this way, you will no longer be angry or green with envy; instead, you will find yourself feeling hopeful and you will look radiant in the color of new growth and rebirth!

Wearing red clothing and accessories helps to support your Heart energy, especially in the **summertime.** The Heart is the primary source of warming energy for the entire body, and the summer—with its long sunny days—is the season that replenishes this energy. Red's firepower can also be used during other times of the year to help balance the warm energies of the Heart. Many people love to wear its more robust shades in the coldest of weather and, of course, on such holidays as Valentine's Day when they wish to stoke the flames of passion.

Wearing yellow clothing and accessories lends strong support to the Spleen's energy, especially in **late summer,** *which is the last month of the summer, defined in North America as the month of August.* The color's bright, warm energies help to dry up the Dampness that is prevalent during this time, protecting the Spleen's Qi from becoming too sluggish. Again, this color can be worn anytime of the year if there has been heavy rainfall and your Spleen needs added nurturing as a result.

Wearing white clothing and accessories provides much support to the energy of the Lungs, especially in the **fall.** This may sound shocking to those of you who have been a slave to the *no white after Labor Day* rule; however, it's true. A crisp white shirt or silk scarf will look nice against all the colors typically worn in autumn and will be especially helpful to your Lungs, ensuring that you breathe well despite the Dry air of the fall. Let this be the year that wearing white helps you avoid seasonal allergies and what you thought was the "inevitable" cold or flu.

Wearing black is ideal anytime because it supports your Kidney energy, but it is especially helpful in the **winter.** This is the time of year when your Kidneys need protection from the cold, so make sure you have enough black basics in your closet during these months. It really helps provide the tender loving care these organs crave at this time of year. Black, just like the element of Water, cleanses you of fear, calms your nervous energy, and instills confidence. Have you ever wondered why it's the color people wear most often when they want to look powerful? Or why celebrities are draped in it when they attend galas and award ceremonies? It exudes self-assurance and, given its association with the organ that fuels our fertility, it quite appropriately exudes sex appeal too.

Please bear in mind that while each of the colors discussed here help their corresponding organs deal with the prevailing conditions of a specific season, you should feel free to wear these colors whenever you feel their related organs or emotions need further support, no matter what time of year it is. Embracing color's energy often and effectively enough will enable you to intuitively gravitate toward the hues that heal their associated organs whenever they're in trouble.

Mix up the colors of your home décor:

Purchase different throw pillows, hand towels, or sheets for your home and rotate them according to the seasons—shades of cyan in the spring, shades of red in the summer, shades of yellow in the late summer, white in the fall, and black in the winter. It's the ideal pick-me-up for your physical *and* emotional health, easing the transition many people feel between seasons.

Organ and Color Correlations at a Glance

PRIMARY ORGAN	Liver	Heart	Spleen	Lungs	Kidneys
PARTNER ORGAN	Gallbladder	Small Intestine	Stomach	Large Intestine	Urinary Bladder
COLOR	Cyan (Green and Blue)	Red	Yellow	White	Black
SEASON	Spring	Summer	Late Summer	Fall	Winter

THE FIVE TASTES

Chinese medicine also associates certain tastes with certain organs. Luckily for us, nurturing our health can be a flavorful experience too!

Sour foods in proper amounts increase helpful energy to the Liver and Gallbladder. Their astringent quality works to maintain the balance of fluids in your body, preventing excessive sweating, frequent urination, and diarrhea.

Bitter foods in proper amounts increase helpful energy to the Heart and Small Intestine. They can rid the body of excess Heat and Dampness, and can help alleviate coughing and wheezing, constipation, and fever. Often people confuse bitter- and sour-tasting foods, but your tongue knows the difference. The taste buds on the back of your tongue identify and respond to bitter foods, while the taste buds on the sides of your tongue identify and respond to sour ones. Raw cocoa, tea, and the zest of certain citrus fruits are bitter, whereas the acidic pulp and juices of lemons, grapes, and melon are often sour.

Sweet foods in proper amounts increase helpful energy to the Spleen and Stomach. In Chinese medicine, sweet foods are classified as carbohydrates, including simple sugars, complex starches, pectin, and polysaccharides, as well as proteins. They range from grains such as glutinous rice to mildly sweet meat such as beef. Note that they do *not* mean refined sugars. Sweet foods supplement *Qi* and blood, neutralize the toxic effects of other foods, and help to reduce pain. They also lubricate and sustain the body.

Pungent foods in proper amounts help increase energy to the Lungs and Large Intestine. They work to improve the circulation and the distribution of *Qi*, blood, and nutrients throughout the body.

Salty foods in proper amounts help increase energy to the Kidneys and Urinary Bladder. They prevent energy stagnation by dissolving the buildup of mucus and soft masses in the body. They also nourish the blood, increase waste elimination, and reduce constipation. Despite these benefits, this is *not* an invitation to overindulge. Many of us love the taste of salty foods as much as we love sugary ones and have been told for years by Western doctors that they are not good for us, so learning of these benefits may falsely encourage some people to add too much salt to their diet. But remember, moderation is the key to all healthy eating.

This discussion raises an extremely important point: **Chinese medicine should not be used the same way that supplements are used in modern medicine.** Very often, Americans hear that something is good for them and they immediately begin to take supplements or eat foods rich in those vitamins or minerals in concentrated forms for an indefinite period of time—sometimes for years! Since all of Chinese medicine is predicated on restoring the body's function to achieve balance, it teaches that doctors should periodically reevaluate their patient's progress and modify the herbal remedies they prescribed based on any changes that subsequently occur in the patient's energy status. Once the goal is achieved, the patient should maintain the newly restored balance through diet, sleep, and such self-care measures as acupressure and qigong. All Chinese herbal supplements prescribed should be monitored by a trained Chinese herbalist. Continuing to take the same herbs in the same doses after balance has been achieved will cause the pendulum to swing in the opposite direction and result in a problem with the opposing organ or energy. An example of this behavior exists in how Americans, based on the recommendation of modern doctors, have added so much omega-3 fatty acids to their diets in an effort to ensure a healthier Heart that many of them have now caused a disruption in the balance of omega-3 to omega-6. Omega-6 is an equally important component of health contributing to brain and muscle development, immune response, fluid retention, and the overall well-being of the central nervous system in our bodies.

What you will find next are general recommendations for tastes and their corresponding food sources to blend into your diet as the seasons—and the respective Qi they generate—change. Should you detect a more noticeable imbalance in the energy of any single organ than what naturally occurs with the passing of the seasons, seek the help of a Chinese medicine practitioner who can help balance that organ's energy with you, overseeing and monitoring its response to the introduction of specific herbs, fruits, vegetables, and meats. Please don't try to self-prescribe tonics!

EASY THINGS YOU CAN DO USING TASTE TO NURTURE YOUR ORGANS

Generally include some sour foods in your diet during the **springtime** when Wind Qi tends to disperse your Liver energy. **Lemons, dark plums, green peppers, string beans, zucchini, mung and lima beans, spinach, collards, green onions, green grapes, green olives, vinegar, and kiwi** are just a few examples of sour foods that can help balance and restore Liver Qi and calm the whole body.

Add some bitter foods to your diet during the **summer** months when Heat Qi can sometimes cause your blood to overheat, and your Heart and Stomach to need some further aid and protection. **Asparagus, bitter melon, arugula, wild cucumber, celery, endives, grapefruit, cranberries, kale, dark chocolate, watercress, parsley, aloe, turmeric, dill, radish, cilantro, eggplant, chamomile,**

basil, barley, okra, blackberries, amaranth, red lentil, sunflower seeds, pistachios, and sage are all helpful to your Heart.

Indulge your taste buds in some sweet foods during the **late summer** season when Damp *Qi* requires that your Spleen get some extra love and care. I know this goes against your every instinct, but trust me, even sweet foods, as long as they are not refined sugars, offer health benefits at the right time and in the right amounts.

Some mildly sweet foods that best aid the Spleen in digesting and absorbing nutrients include **carrots, sweet potatoes, parsnips, rutabagas, squash, figs, onions, chickpeas, cinnamon, oranges, papaya, pineapples, strawberries, pine nuts, pumpkins, peas, zucchini, apples, bananas, bok choy, fresh ginger, beets, coconut, chestnuts, lychee, spelt, leeks, endives, fava beans, and honey**.

Many Americans are most conscious of their appearance during the late summer months—the height of bathing suit season and the time of year when they are wearing the most revealing clothing. During this season they tend to increase their intake of raw foods such as fruits, salads, and juices, thinking that these are the healthiest of choices. However, this is counterintuitive as these moisture-packed foods can increase Damp *Qi* in your system, which often causes bloating and slows down your metabolism. Enjoy some of the sweet foods listed here instead and you will be doing your summer figure a great favor.

Incorporate a few pungent foods in your diet during the **fall** to keep your Lungs healthy in the Dry air and your Large Intestine functioning smoothly. Some pungent foods include **ginger, garlic, asparagus, broccoli, mustard greens, onion, radish, apricot, banana, pear, almonds, navy beans, soy, rice, turnips, lotus seeds, cauliflower, peaches, oregano, anise, chili, chives, kale, and chard**.

Lastly, spice things up with some naturally salty foods during the **winter** months to boost your Kidneys and direct the flow of excess water through your Urinary Bladder—but do so in moderation. You will recall that black-colored foods are also energetically helpful to the Kidneys. Foods you should enjoy include **azuki** beans, black beans, kidney beans, millet, barley, buckwheat, black sesame seeds, flax, walnuts, chives, leeks, wheatgrass, asparagus, dark-green leafy vegetables, parsley, black mushrooms, seaweeds, abalone, crab, clams, sea cucumber, oysters, mussels, sardines, octopus, shrimp, mulberry, pomegranate, raspberry, watermelon, water chestnut, cherries, black rice, bone-marrow broth, and sea salt. These foods will add to the luster of your hair as well.

By the way, you will note that some of the foods recommended in this section differ from those recommended for each organ in prior chapters. Fortunately, life is a feast—many different foods can be counted on to provide the same kinds of nutritional values, all while keeping the palate fresh. Consider the foods mentioned earlier as staples for each organ. These newly added foods aid your organs at different times of the year and under different conditions. **Remember that the energy of each organ is constantly changing in accordance with the energies introduced to it from the environment. The foods recommended in this chapter are all intended to help restore balance whenever the seasons tip the scales and create a bit of havoc with that balance!** The more you become in tune with your body, the easier it will be for you to keep track of what to eat and when to eat it. In the meantime, you can easily refer to this book for quick tips and the Seasonal Shopping List provided in chapter 11.

Organ and Taste Correlations at a Glance

PRIMARY ORGAN	Liver	Heart	Spleen	Lungs	Kidneys
PARTNER ORGAN	Gallbladder	Small Intestine	Stomach	Large Intestine	Urinary Bladder
TASTE	Sour	Bitter	Sweet	Pungent	Salty
SEASON	Spring	Summer	Late Summer	Fall	Winter

THE FIVE SOUNDS

Chinese medicine also teaches us that sound can have a positive effect on our health.

One of the most nurturing things you can do for yourself is listen to a live classical music performance. Every year, I take my family and a few friends to see Shen Yun Performing Arts, a classical Chinese dance troupe accompanied by a full orchestra that combines both Western and traditional Chinese instrumentation. The effect of this music is so powerful that all of my guests tell me they feel recharged after the experience. Many times I can see their faces begin to relax and transform right in front of me. They look more youthful already—carefree and joyful.

Music is considered so healing and therapeutic in Chinese culture that practitioners of Chinese medicine regularly use it to treat a wide range of illnesses. In fact, the traditional character for medicine in the Chinese language includes the character for music.

It was *Huang Di Nei Jing* that first revealed this connection between music and health. Since that time much proof has been gathered to support the fact that each of the five tones in the most common scale in Chinese music—the five-tone pentatonic scale—corresponds with a different human organ, helping to nurture and balance the energy of that organ. In Chinese, these five tones are called *gōng* (宮), *shāng* (商), *jué* (角), *zhǐ* (徵), and *yǔ* (羽), but every fan of the movie *The Sound of Music* knows them as do, re, mi, so, and la. This scale can be very soothing because it has no half-tones, which are the tones that typically create tension in a piece.

Gōng or do: A musical piece with *gōng* as the major tone tends to be peaceful, steady, soft, and smooth. Like the earth, it nurtures and embraces life.

Gōng empowers the energy of the Spleen, which in partnership with the Stomach, is in charge of digestion, metabolism, and energy production. The Spleen nurtures the muscles and prevents bruising and bleeding. It also improves our thinking and our ability to process information; thus music with a lot of *gōng* is good for people who tend to be nervous, bruise easily, have a slow metabolism or poor digestion, or are prone to fatigue. It also helps soothe worry and enhances compassion.

This kind of music is wonderful to listen to year-round, but it is especially supportive in the late summer.

An example of *gōng* music can be found in the piece "Ambushed from Ten Sides." This is one of ten ancient classic pieces in Chinese musical history. The composer is unknown.

Shāng or re: The sound of *shāng* is harmonious, nurturing, pure, and clear. *Shāng* empowers the energy of the Lungs. In partnership with the Large Intestine, the Lungs are in charge of breathing and the distribution of vital energy to the entire body through blood vessels and energy channels.

The Lungs also nurture the skin and hair, help regulate absorption and elimination of water, and defend the body from external pathogenic energy.

Again, the emotion associated with the Lungs is grief. Therefore, music with the sound of *shāng* is good for people who are mourning or sad, those who easily catch colds, and those who have problems with their sinuses and respiratory system.

Music with *shāng* can help empower you when you feel mentally weak, and it also enhances a sense of loyalty and control.

This kind of music is wonderful to listen to year-round, but it is especially supportive in the fall.

An example of music with the tone *shāng* can be found in "White Snow in Early Spring." This is also one of the ten ancient classics. It is believed to have been composed by Shi Kuang or Liu Zejuan in the spring or autumn, between 771 and 476 B.C.

Jué or mi: The sound of *jué* is youthful, uplifting, and full of life. It reaches high and far and moves up and down smoothly and continuously.

The tone of *jué* empowers the energy of the Liver, which, in partnership with the Gallbladder, is in charge of the free flow of the energy and blood, and regulates digestion, menstruation, moods, and sleep.

Therefore, music with *jué* is good for people who are depressed or irritable or have headaches, pain, insomnia, and high blood pressure.

Jué also helps with strategic planning and judgment; soothes anger, resentment, and frustration; and helps vision. It can also strengthen tolerance and kindness.

This kind of music is wonderful to listen to year-round, but it is especially supportive in the spring.

An example of music with the *jué* tone can be found in "18 Songs of Nomad Flute." It too is one of the ten ancient classics. It was composed by Cai Wenji between A.D. 25 and 222, during the Eastern Han Dynasty.

Zhǐ or so: The sound of *zhǐ* is passionate, ascending, and gracefully joyful. *Zhǐ* empowers the energy of the Heart, which, in partnership with the Small Intestine, is in charge of the higher functions of the central nervous system, including cognition, sensory perception, and language.

The Heart also nurtures the blood vessels and helps improve the complexion of the face.

Music with *zhǐ* is good for people with poor blood circulation, heart problems, and depression, and if the body is cold, music with the *zhǐ* tone helps warm it.

Listening to music with *zhǐ* can also enhance feelings of humility and respect.

This kind of music is wonderful to listen to year-round, but it is especially supportive in the summer.

An example of music with *zhǐ* can be found in the song "Higher Step by Step." This is a lovely piece by modern composer Lui Wencheng.

Yǔ or la: The sound of *yǔ* is powerful and purifying, like a waterfall high up on a tall mountain.

Yǔ empowers the energy of the Kidneys, which, in partnership with the Bladder, are in charge of absorption and elimination of water, as well as the energy that nurtures the brain, bones, and hair.

The Kidneys also oversee sexual function and conception, and aid in our hearing as well.

Music with *yǔ* is good for people who want to improve self-control, physical agility, fertility, intelligence, memory, and concentration. It also strengthens the mind's willpower and dispels fear. Lastly, it is known to make people feel generous.

This kind of music is wonderful to listen to year-round, but it is especially supportive in the winter.

An example of music with *yǔ* can be found in "Autumn Moon over Han Palace." Like several of the other recommended pieces, this is one of the ten famous ancient classics. Its composer is unknown.

When selecting music to help balance your *Qi*, remember that from the Chinese medicine perspective, traditional or classical music is best. In the same way that harmonious music can soothe and heal your body, disharmonious music can be unsettling and harmful.

MORE EASY THINGS YOU CAN DO USING SOUND TO NURTURE YOUR ORGANS

After listening to the suggested music, improve your health and broaden your cultural awareness even more by seeking out other forms of world music that utilize the calming tones of the pentatonic scale. Pandora, Spotify, Beats, and other streaming services can help you expand your search.

Add songs to your playlist that are associated with happy memories and listen to them often.

Share your new music discoveries with others. We contend with so much noise pollution in our day-to-day lives that sending more soothing sounds into the world may help balance more than just our own energy. And when at home, try listening to comforting music without your earbuds or headphones every once in a while. Let your environment absorb these nurturing sounds too, as long as the volume remains at a respectable level.

Organ and Phonetics Correlations at a Glance

PRIMARY ORGAN	Liver	Heart	Spleen	Lungs	Kidneys
PARTNER ORGAN	Gallbladder	Small Intestine	Stomach	Large Intestine	Urinary Bladder
PHONETICS	Mi	So	Do	Re	La
SEASON	Spring	Summer	Late Summer	Fall	Winter

THE FIVE SEASONS

I hope that by now you see the clear connections that exist between these group-ings of five and their respective organs, as well as the connections each of these groups have to one another. This is how the world is viewed through the prism of Chinese medicine. All things exist in relationship to something else—often in rela-tionship to many other things! **Maintaining balance between all these elements is how energy remains vibrant, in constant motion, and in continual service to the repair and regeneration of all matter.** Essentially, it's how energy maintains life itself. How it keeps you healthy, vital, and looking fresher than your actual years would indicate.

If you look closely at the preceding sections of this chapter, you will see how effec-tively you can manage your health and beauty each season by using the many valuable tools at your disposal including elements, color, taste, and sound, among many other factors still to be discovered in this book. When used properly and in concert with each other, they can truly help you fine-tune the balance between the internal and external energies that continue to cycle around us. In summary:

The spring is associated with the Liver. Spring is the time when everything is
renewing and regenerating. Likewise, it is the time when the Liver renews and

regenerates the body. In spring, Wind is the predominant energy that keeps everything moving outside of us, just as the Liver *Qi* is the energy that keeps everything moving inside our bodies. Because the Liver is sensitive to Wind, it must be particularly well nurtured throughout the spring's gusty months. Woodsy elements, the blend of green and blue we call the color cyan, sour-tasting foods, and the mi tone all help the Liver *Qi* achieve harmony.

The summer is associated with the Heart. Summer is the time when everything develops more completely. The Heart is what helps us develop more fully too—physically, mentally, and spiritually. The predominant energy in the summer is Heat. This Heat warms the planet just as the Heart warms our body. Because the Heart is sensitive to Heat, it must be particularly well nurtured throughout the summer's hot months. The element of Fire, the color red, bitter-tasting foods, and the so tone all have the potential to help keep the Heart *Qi* in balance.

The late summer is associated with the Spleen. Late summer, which we recognize as the month of August, is a transformative time just as the Spleen is a transformative organ. The Spleen converts what we eat and drink into *Postnatal Jing*. The strongest energy in late summer is Dampness. Because the Spleen is sensitive to Dampness, it must be particularly well nurtured throughout late summer's sultry and humid months. The element of Earth, the color yellow, sweet-tasting foods, and the do tone all help the Spleen *Qi* remain balanced.

The fall is associated with the Lungs. Fall is the season of harvesting, when everything is mature and ready to be gathered and stored. The Lungs are where the *Qi* is formed and distributed, combining both *Prenatal* and *Postnatal Qi*. Dryness is the major energy in fall. Because the Lungs are sensitive to Dryness, they must be particularly well nurtured throughout the fall's arid months. The element of Metal, pungent-tasting foods, the color white, and the re tone all help the Lung *Qi* remain balanced.

The winter is associated with the Kidneys. Winter is the time of conservation, when nature goes into retreat. The principal energy in winter is coldness.

The Kidneys provide Cold energy in the body to balance the Heat energy emanating from the Heart. Because the Kidneys are sensitive to Cold, they must be particularly well nurtured throughout the winter's frigid months. The element of Water, the color black, salty-tasting foods, and the la tone all help Kidney Qi remain balanced.

As promised earlier, the following is a comprehensive chart commonly used in the understanding and practice of classical Chinese medicine. It illustrates how all of the factors we've discussed so far (and many others still to be discussed) work in tandem to maintain the health of the body, mind, and spirit. Reviewing each column will help you remember how to readily nurture each organ in several different ways during the months when that organ is most vulnerable—and at any other time during the year when it may need extra care! We will refer to this chart frequently in the pages ahead. Trust that your grasp of its meaning and applications will deepen each time.

THE THEORY OF FIVE ELEMENTS SUMMARY CHART

ELEMENT	Wood	Fire	Earth	Metal	Water
PRIMARY ORGAN	Liver	Heart	Spleen	Lungs	Kidneys
PARTNER ORGAN	Gallbladder	Small Intestine	Stomach	Large Intestine	Urinary Bladder
EMOTION	Anger	Joy	Worry	Grief	Fear
COLOR	Cyan	Red	Yellow	White	Black
TASTE	Sour	Bitter	Sweet	Pungent	Salty
SEASON	Spring	Summer	Late Summer	Fall	Winter
ENERGY	Wind	Heat	Dampness	Dryness	Cold
SENSORY ORGAN AND SENSE	Eyes Vision	Tongue Speech	Mouth Taste	Nose Smell	Ears Hearing
RELATED ORGANS	Tendons, Ligaments	Pulse, Veins, Arteries	Muscles, Flesh	Skin	Bones, Joints
EXTERNAL MANIFES- TATION	Nails	Complexion	Lips	Body Hair	Head Hair
BODY FLUID	Tears	Sweat	Saliva	Mucus	Urine
PHONETICS	Mi	So	Do	Re	La
FUNCTION	Generating	Developing	Transforming	Harvesting	Conserving
PHYSICAL FUNCTIONS	Digestion, Qi Movement, Menstruation, Sleep	Blood Vessels, Circulation	Immune System, Digestion, Absorption, Metabolism, Blood Containment (to prevent bleeding)	Breathing, Water Passage	Growth, Development, Reproduction, Sexual Function

SPIRITUAL AND MENTAL FUNCTIONS	Hun (The Ethereal Soul) Vision, Decision Making, Strategy, Judgment	Shen (The Emperor of the Soul) Consciousness, Perception, Cognition, Emotion, Language, Initiative	Yi (The Mindful Soul) Thoughts, Ideas, Intention, Reasoning	Po (The Corporal Soul) Mental Discipline, Order, Sensitivity, Restraint	Zhi (The Willful Soul) Motivation, Determination, Willpower, Coordination
MENTAL QUALITY	Sensitivity	Creativity	Clarity	Intuition	Spontaneity
SOUND	Shouting	Laughing	Singing	Crying	Moaning
SMELL	Rancid or Foul	Burnt	Sweet or Fragrant	Rank or Fishy	Putrid
SIGN OF ILLNESS	Exhibiting Logorrhea	Belching	Slurring	Coughing	Yawning
GRAINS AND VEGETABLES	Wheat, Mallow	Beans, Greens	Rice, Scallions	Corn, Onions	Millet, Leeks

Norma's Musings on Sensory Awareness

If you really want to witness how the environment affects you and how you affect the environment, take a walk in a designer's shoes for a day. Fashion designers have to produce a new line every season—that means coming up with lots of fresh yet viable ideas four times a year and seeing them to fruition. To do that, we have to have our sensors on all the time. We see things constantly that many other people miss simply because they're not actively looking. We're observing every second to gather information and inspiration. This behavior becomes automatic. I've spent my whole life viewing things, capturing them, and letting them register in the same way I take a breath.

My senses are particularly heightened when I travel. And I am fortunate enough to travel a lot. When I was younger, I had a job at an airline selling tours so I could take off every weekend to a different locale, although I enjoyed going to London more often than anywhere else. It was a burgeoning time culturally, and London in particular was ushering in exciting new fashions, music, art, and changing social and political views. To this day I still travel for pleasure as well as for business. On my birthday each year, a friend who is an astrologer suggests a place for me to visit that my chart indicates is auspicious for personal growth. I never know where it's going to be. It's always an adventure. Some places are better for me than others and I can feel my health shift in response. There are places where my energies feel incompatible and other places where I am just buzzing, taking everything in and feeling completely energized, excited, curious, inspired, and in sync with my surroundings. My first trip to China was like that. It was beyond anything I could have imagined. It's a place where you can see a clear future for the next generation. It's radiating vibrant energy right now, like a supernova. There is a sense of unharnessed potential but also a cultural understanding of all the greatness of the past, and of how to bring that greatness forward in the most modern and relevant ways. It's an energy that drew me in in the same way that the energy of London in the 1960s did.

In many respects this intersection of the old and the new is at the heart of *Yin* and *Yang*, a point in which the two are finding balance in transformation.

I have always believed that what makes a person truly beautiful is feeling alive. Setting yourself in a place that speaks energetically to your senses is one of the best ways to invigorate yourself and jumpstart your personal inner and outer revitalization. Going to China is what made me want to pursue and embrace acupuncture. It's what introduced me to new health and beauty concepts to add to those I was already practicing. It was ultimately what set me off on this project with Dr. Yang. To enjoy similar experiences of revitalization, take a trip to somewhere new or resolve to play tourist in your own city for a day, paying closer attention to your surroundings than usual. Find the things around you that excite you, that make you want to step into the day, or that bring you comfort and peace at the end of the night. Take in the colors, the sounds, and the tastes and see how they affect you physically, spiritually, and emotionally. I love that the color of the sky is dramatically different in New York City than it is in Beijing or Florence. I also love that some sun-drenched places make me want to abandon my urban camouflage and just wear colors that reflect the vibrant yellows and oranges around me. That's what happens when I'm in India, for instance.

When we are very young—before the influences of fashion, our jobs, the weather, or the city we live in take hold—we have this kind of pure relationship with the outside world. It's especially noticeable with regard to color. At age three or four, we gravitate toward the ones that fuel our energy and also reflect our energies back to the world. But when we grow up, we tend to seek out the colors that help us navigate our daily surroundings better. In a city like New York we wear defense colors. Only when we want to call attention to ourselves, rather than blend in, do we veer away from black, gray, and other neutrals. For example, when we are at the gym and want to show off our hard-earned physique, some of us might add a pop of green to our workout clothes. So when you walk around either a new or familiar environment today, try to connect with it as innocently as a child would. Note the things that energize, inspire, calm, or soothe you. Really pay attention to them as if you were encountering them for the first time. Then consciously reintroduce some of those same sights, sounds, and colors into your home and life so they can stoke or reflect your natural energies once again.

2

Your Body

5

Getting Ahead of the Aging Process

SECRETS TO HEALTHY AND BEAUTIFUL HAIR

NK It's been extremely helpful to learn about all the different factors our internal organs are exposed to—those that disrupt our energies and age us, as well as those that have the amazing power to promote healing. **I wonder if we can look more closely now at the *visible* signs of aging so we can discover ways to slow, halt, or even *reverse* them if that is possible?**

JY Yes, of course. The visible signs of aging are what bring most patients to my door every day. It's human nature. We don't always pay attention to what's going on inside of us, but when it starts to show up on the outside for everyone else to see, that's when we know we have to act to correct it. I don't think this behavior of ours is vanity so much as a sudden awareness of something not being the way it used to be. The good news is that while signs of aging seem to sneak up on many of us almost overnight, signs of improvement can be relatively quick to develop, too, if you follow the rules.

Let's do a thorough examination from head to toe together, beginning with our hair.

In ancient China, long hair was a symbol of longevity. Hair is an inherited trait from one's parents so you didn't dare cut it—that would be like cutting ties with those who gave you life. So over time, the length of your hair suggested how old you were. The association between hair, longevity, and the source of life was only deepened by the teachings of Chinese medicine. It tells us that our hair is nurtured by the Kidneys, which oversee reproduction and fertility as well as the storage and distribution of *Jing,* the essence of *Qi* and life itself. Although hairstyles in China have changed dramatically since ancient times and people feel free to cut their hair as frequently as they like, Chinese people typically take very good care of their hair to this day. Understanding the connection between your hair and your Kidneys can help you take better care of your hair as well.

You can trace the roots of your hair's health back to the Kidneys in a different way, too. When you are having your hair washed at the salon, that tingling feeling you get is not only your nerve endings being invigorated. It's the circulation of blood beneath the scalp. Every day your blood delivers nutrients to your hair. The Spleen and Stomach send these nutrients from the foods you eat, but your blood is also fortified in the bone marrow by the *Prenatal Jing* stored in your Kidneys. For you to have healthy hair you must keep both your Blood *Qi* and your Kidney *Qi* healthy. That means eating a balanced diet filled with foods that nurture your Blood and Kidney essence. It also means making sure that you conserve your *Prenatal Jing.*

One way to do this is to rethink the popular American saying "Use it or lose it." This saying is actually the opposite of what Chinese medicine believes. Living every day at a fast pace will only consume your *Jing* or life force and leave you without enough *Qi* to support your primary organs and the other visible organs associated with them. It's one reason why young people get gray hair too (even if only they and their hair colorist know about it!). **It is not that age affects our Kidneys and in turn our hair; it's that the poor care of our Kidneys causes us to age both inside and out.**

Of course, while lifestyle is a major factor in our hair's appearance, it is not the only one. If you live moderately and make healthy choices, yet still have hair issues, it may very well be that your parents used up a significant portion of their *Prenatal Jing* in their youth and were unable to genetically pass it along to you in a greater quantity when you were born. In this case, it is especially important for you to bolster your *Postnatal Jing* through proper diet. You should be evaluated to assess what other possible impacts deficient Kidney *Jing* and *Qi* may be having on your health as well. And be sure to ask your practitioner to provide a meal plan to help you make up for what you are missing nutritionally.

Another factor that contributes to unhealthy hair is excessive Heat in one's blood. This can cause your hair to become dry and brittle and to fall out. People should avoid consuming alcohol as well as fatty or spicy foods and opt instead for cooling foods if this is an issue for them.

If you're still not sure that your allotment of *Jing* and the health of your Kidneys are somehow connected to the health of your hair, consider an unusual experience I had when I was in medical school. While studying modern medicine, I learned that the blood is produced in the bone marrow, but all the texts I had ever read about Chinese medicine said it is Kidney essence that produces blood. So imagine how surprised I was to learn that in 1952 Dr. Allan J. Erslev, who later became director of the Cardeza Foundation of Hematologic Research at Jefferson Medical College, now called Sidney Kimmel Medical College, where I currently work, discovered a hormone called erythropoietin, which is produced by the Kidney in order to help stimulate the bone marrow to produce blood. This hormone is presently being synthesized as a treatment for patients undergoing chemotherapy so they can manage the fluctuations in their blood cell count. Modern medicine, in this case, supplied the missing link that explained an assertion made by Chinese medicine centuries ago. Given my knowledge of Chinese medicine, I began to wonder if this hormone that is produced by the Kidneys and helps stimulate the blood—and is also very likely to be part of what we know as Kidney *Jing*—could be used to nurture every other function in the body served by the Kidneys as we understand them in classical Chinese medicine. Logic suggests that it should not only be able to improve the quality of your hair, it should be able to support your brainpower too—particularly your cognitive functions, motivation, and willpower! It should also be able to help you maintain your bone health, staving off osteoporosis. And, of course, it should even help sexual function and fertility. I thought I had struck gold. So I looked through a variety of medical journals to see if anyone else was exploring these possibilities. Guess what? Some studies had already been done! There was a published paper stating that this hormone did in fact improve cognitive function in mice. It is now being used to help patients suffering from depression too. I imagine that it works very much like Kidney *Jing* does in reducing patients' fears and increasing their willpower. This is just one example of the many ways breakthroughs in modern medicine are supporting age-old theories practiced in Chinese medicine for more than 2,500 years.

To help you preserve your *Prenatal Jing*, boost your *Postnatal Jing*, keep your blood vibrant and healthy, and restore luster to your hair, let me recount some of the tips we talked about earlier and add several more in the next section.

A FEW EASY STEPS YOU CAN TAKE TO HELP NURTURE YOUR HAIR

Rid yourself of fear, because fear blocks and diminishes your Kidney energy. You will discover a particularly effective technique in chapter 8 to help you banish this difficult emotion, but until then, take deep cleansing breaths, focus on the here and now, and tap or massage your Kidney 1 and Kidney 3 points along your Kidney Meridian to help stir your *Qi*'s movement as illustrated on page 83.

Manage your sex life to help minimize the loss of *Jing*. Men should be aware that their *Jing* escapes every time they ejaculate. Practicing seminal retention from time to time can help. If you are a woman, be sure to rest and eat properly during your menstrual cycle, particularly if your blood flow tends to be heavy. It is also wise to replenish your body in the months following childbirth and during the time you spend breast-feeding. Giving birth depletes a fair amount of a woman's blood supply, and she also shares her supply of *Prenatal Jing* with her baby. Since breast-feeding requires her to pass along many of the nutrients she gains from her food intake to her child, she must eat sufficiently to increase her *Postnatal Jing* as well.

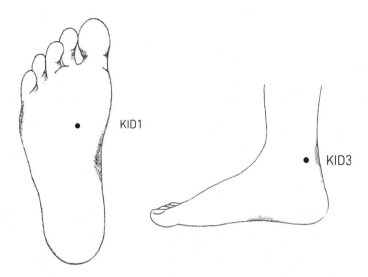

Eat foods that nurture your Kidneys, including grains, cooked dark-green leafy
    vegetables, black mushrooms, black soybeans, black sesame seeds, walnuts,
    chestnuts, and dark fruits.

Add Kidney-nourishing herbs such as ginseng and rehmannia root to your diet.

In the winter months when your Kidneys need a little more care, add a few salty
    foods to your diet, including soybean paste (made from fermented soybean) or
    soy sauce, fish, shrimp, and seaweed, or use a pinch more sea salt when cooking.

Gently massage your Kidney area twice daily—once in the morning and once in
    the evening—for fifteen minutes each time. Rub your palms together thirty-six
    times to warm your hands before doing so.

Also be sure to get sufficient sleep, especially in winter. During those months
    you should go to bed earlier than usual and grant yourself permission to
    wake up late too. Remember that your blood and your Kidneys are nurtured
    while you rest!

Comb or brush your hair daily. Use a wooden comb or a black-bristle brush.
    Start from the back midline of your head and stroke from the root of your
    hair to the very ends of your hair, making sure that your scalp feels the

sensation too. As you do this, you will be stroking the parietal, the occipital, and finally the neck regions. Be sure that you brush one hundred times. Then repeat this same process on the sides and lateral parts of your head. Your head is where all *Yang* energy channels meet. It has more than forty acupuncture points and many more areas where stimulation has proven beneficial. Combing these points will help your energy and blood circulate better. It will also calm you and improve your memory and concentration as well as your vision, hearing, bone health, and overall well-being. Radiant hair is, of course, an incredible bonus!

If you believe your hair loss is due more to lack of blood circulation than to dryness, massage your scalp with thin slices of ginger for ten to fifteen minutes a day. Ginger's generating qualities can help your blood circulate and rejuvenate cell growth.

After shampooing, wrap your hair in a black towel to help restore energy while the hair dries.

Wear black clothing, particularly on the lower half of your body and during the winter months.

Place a black lumbar pillow on your office chair to support your Kidneys while you work.

Listen to meditative music or hum the la tone of the pentatonic scale to yourself in the shower.

Swallow your own saliva several times a day. It is very good for your Kidney energy and therefore for all of the organs along the Kidney Meridian, including your hair. Close your mouth slightly and, starting above your teeth, sweep your tongue around clockwise for twelve cycles; then repeat this process twelve times in the counterclockwise direction. While Chinese medicine has known the benefits of saliva for centuries, modern medicine has more recently confirmed that it contains a combination of antimicrobial agents, enzymes, antibodies, and even an analgesic in addition to cell-growth properties.

PATIENT-TESTED TRUTHS

Here I must stop and tell you the remarkable story of a thirty-four-year-old patient named Joy who had a hard time living up to her name as she struggled with chronic lower back pain and anxiety marked by fear and lack of motivation. When we first met, there was no detectable abnormality in her lumbar spine and she was responding poorly to medications intended to treat her back pain and mood. Chinese medicine, however, understands that this condition stems from the stagnation of *Qi* in the Kidney and Bladder channels. This stagnation typically causes deficiency and blocks the free flow of Kidney *Jing* to the brain and bone marrows, preventing them from being properly nurtured. With the aid of ongoing acupuncture treatments, Kidney *Jing* and *Qi* tonics, as well as dietary changes to support her Kidneys and to supply additional nourishment to the bone marrow, Joy's chronic lower back pain and anxiety virtually disappeared, much to the shock of her modern doctors. It took several more months, but after her lower back pain and anxiety were resolved, Joy also reported that her hair, which was noticeably thinning, dry, and brittle before treatment, was now growing back quickly and was fuller than ever, proving once again the interconnectivity of our outer appearance and inner health and the specific connection between our Kidneys, blood circulation, and hair.

MY PERSONAL SECRET TO A GOOD HAIR DAY

I have one final suggestion to help your hair look and feel as silky, soft, vibrant, natural, voluminous, and most of all as healthy as you would like. It comes directly from the recipes of the royal kitchen.

In China people eat congee the way Americans eat cereal or oatmeal. It is a rice-based porridge that is simple and easy to make. Depending on the ingredients you add, mothers and practitioners of Chinese medicine agree that it can cure a lot of what ails you and keep you looking young for a very, very long time. Here is one of the congee recipes I grew up eating, particularly during the wintertime. It is intended to help fortify your hair.

Congee Recipe for Beautiful Hair
(MAKES 4 SERVINGS)

INGREDIENTS:

½ cup of rice

4 cups of water

1 cup of walnuts

½ cup of black sesame seeds

Wash rice thoroughly. Put the rice and the water in a pot and bring to a boil over medium heat. Reduce heat to a simmer and cover.

Reserve a few walnuts and sesame seeds for toppings, then grind the rest into a powder.

When the rice is 70 percent cooked and the remaining water is still rich and creamy, add the powder and stir for one minute.

Serve hot with the nut and seed garnish.

Try it and see what wonders it works!

Norma's Musings on Healthy Hair and What Is Still a Gray Area for Many Women: To Color or Not to Color?

I'm a great experimenter. I always have been. I love change. I know that for a lot of people, change is disturbing and disarming. It makes them feel insecure and nervous, but I find it forces me to think in new ways. I'm always spontaneously moving everyone's desk around in the office or deciding to work in a different room. All of a sudden it's as if I have a new vantage point. Change provides a fresh way to look at everything. You feel different when you see the world from a new perspective. This is what has helped me reinvent myself a thousand times since I started my career in 1967.

For years I changed my hair color a lot, too. I like for people to see me in a new light from time to time. I loved being a redhead, and I'm fond of my current shade as well. But as much as I like change, and as much I have moved into more natural alternatives in the rest of my beauty regimen, I don't see myself transitioning into gray hair as readily as I've previously transitioned into other looks. Symbolically, in all cultures it defines you chronologically. I love the idea of having long gray strands and bangs with only black tips along the edges. I think it would be gorgeous from a fashion point of view. But what keeps me from doing it—and what has me continuing my efforts to develop a natural solution I can use healthfully to cover whatever gray is coming in—is that gray is a sign that the body is lacking its own color and vitality, and I am feeling the opposite of gray. I am always on the search for healthy colors and look forward to someday finding a solution to the hair-color challenge.

What we can all do to prolong the time we spend as a natural blonde, brunette, or redhead, however, is to really take care of our hair in all the ways Dr. Yang suggests. I absolutely love massages. They are critical to good health. Second only to enjoying a good Thai massage, which is ideal for stretching out the body's muscles, is the ritual of getting an amazing scalp massage. It does wonders for your hair. It gets the blood and Qi flowing to all the right places. A scalp massage is always available at the nearest hair salon but you can give yourself a scalp massage daily as well. Inspire your partner to make scalp massages part of your interaction and share giving them. Also, there is nothing like acupuncture to increase blood and energy flow. My hair and complexion always look really good afterward, so I recommend acupuncture for shiny, healthy hair as well.

Also, be mindful of overwashing your hair and using blow-dryers, curling irons, and other heated tools too much. Nothing makes your hair look old and decrepit more than *dead ends*, so getting a good cut and changing up your style is always a good idea too.

Lastly, I wash with a soap-free shampoo and replenish my body's natural oils through a healthy diet that includes fish and other foods high in omega-3 fatty acids. I also use an olive oil liniment when I want to give my hair a deep conditioning or when I'm spending a day at the beach. My mother used to do this for me, and it is a practice that works to this day. While using olive oil as a conditioner is not something born out of Chinese medicine, I think it is in line with the philosophy. To me, applying olive oil topically is another means of nurturing my body. Including it in my diet is also a means of replenishing my *Postnatal Jing*.

I will reference my love of olive oil a fair amount in the pages to come, so let me just give you a little background. My mother, who is Lebanese, had it in our home at all times. Olive oil can be used as a moisturizer, with a salt scrub, as massage oil—and to keep us regular, in all of our meals, and as a lubricant for lovemaking. Many olive trees are centuries old. They are hearty and have survived the test of time. Therefore olive oil is truly all-purpose and timeless. Doesn't that suggest it would be a good choice to enhance diet and health, and for personal use? I have visited olive orchards in France, Italy, and Spain and carry a collection of some of the purest beauty products made from these oils in my WELLNESS CAFÉ. It is a gift of love I give to my friends each year during the new harvest in November.

6

Doing an About-Face

RETURNING TO A MORE YOUTHFUL COMPLEXION

The other great beauty preoccupation we all have, of course, is with the care of our complexion. This is true throughout all stages of life. We wonder how to keep our skin from being too oily or too dry. How to rid ourselves of blemishes, age spots, hives, rashes, and more. And how to avoid wrinkles altogether. The care of our skin is of particular concern to people who love being outside in the sun. **Dr. Yang, what can you tell our readers that will enable them to naturally maintain, preserve, or rejuvenate their skin?**

Norma makes yet another interesting point. Americans tend to love basking on the beach during the summer months and visiting tanning salons in the wintertime, whereas Chinese people generally shield themselves year-round from the effects of the sun's UV rays. They prize fair skin and wear sun hats and carry parasols for added protection. What they understand is that our facial complexion is often better nurtured with the help of our internal organs than by the sun.

According to Chinese medicine, our complexion is associated with the Heart and its partner, the Small Intestine. Both work to supply nutrient-rich blood to our faces, increasing circulation and giving us that natural blush that's far healthier for us than a tan could ever be.

Again, you can see that when you wish to maintain or restore the health of an outer feature, you must first nurture its corresponding internal organs. In other words, to have wonderful skin you must strive to have a good and strong Heart.

Whether we are looking at the health of your facial skin or for signs that your Heart *Qi* is somehow imbalanced, practitioners of Chinese medicine will begin by focusing on the *evenness* of your complexion. We want to know if your color is consistent. A uniform tone lets us know that your blood is circulating well and that the veins and arteries are free and clear to carry nourishment as far as the tiniest vessels in the outer reaches of the body. Your face is filled with such vessels so it is an excellent measure of your Blood *Qi*'s mobility.

If, instead of an even complexion, we see that you have blotches, breakouts, rosacea, or hives, we know something else is interfering with the consistency and flow of *Qi* along the Heart Meridian. Acne, for instance, signals that Heat, Dampness, and toxins are collecting at the skin level because your Small Intestine is unable to process fats effectively or because it is unable to detoxify the blood. This imbalance keeps the Heart from sending the most nutrient-rich blood to the surface where it would otherwise keep your face looking fresh and invigorated.

By the way, your complexion is an excellent barometer of your Heart's emotional health too. Ever notice how when you are feeling embarrassed, shy, upset, flustered, nervous, or overly excited, you experience a rush of color to your face? Your skin's reaction to these emotions tells us a lot about the condition of your Heart.

In addition to noting the evenness of color, practitioners of Chinese medicine learn a lot from the pallor of your complexion.

- A white pallor indicates deficiency in Blood and *Qi* or excessive *Yin* energy brought about by the Cold.
- A yellow pallor suggests that too much Dampness exists in the blood and that you may have a possible Spleen *Qi* Deficiency. In cases of jaundice, where

excessive Damp Heat impedes your Liver from doing its job properly, the skin (and the eyes) turn a bright orange-yellow. By contrast, a dark yellow cast to the skin suggests the presence of too much Damp Cold.

- Redness suggests that the blood vessels are swelling due to excessive Heat. You'll notice this when you have a fever or are experiencing hot flashes.
- A blue pallor in the face or extremities signals Cold, pain, and/or Blood Stasis. This is a warning sign that *Qi* and blood blockages exist somewhere along the Heart Meridian.
- A black pallor indicates a Kidney *Qi* Deficiency and possible Blood Stasis.

A FEW EASY STEPS YOU CAN TAKE TO HELP NURTURE YOUR COMPLEXION

Each of the scenarios just described requires a specific treatment by an experienced practitioner. However, the following are general suggestions that can help you proactively support your Heart and Small Intestine every day and avoid any potential health challenges in the future while also giving you the natural, radiant complexion you are longing for.

Although I've said it before, it bears repeating: You must first let go of any negative emotional attachments you may have and consciously embrace the joy in your life. The Heart in Chinese medicine functions very much like the brain. It's where we receive and process information as well as receive and generate emotion. All decisions and thoughts come from the Heart. It is our consciousness. So if you don't work to keep a clear and wise Heart, everything else will suffer, and that suffering will be most apparent in the quality of your skin. You will recall my saying earlier that Chinese medicine views the Heart as the emperor of the body. If it is enlightened, smart, rational, and intelligent, everyone else in its path will be happy, safe, and prosperous. If it is a ridiculous tyrant, filled with misgivings and prone to self-indulgence and negative feelings, everyone around it will be in danger. When someone says they "have a broken heart," they mean it. So take care of your Heart by making wise decisions. Think carefully about your choice of foods, partners, friends, pursuits, and actions in general. This, of course, will also preserve the quality of your skin and everything else the emperor oversees.

Reduce hot and spicy foods in your diet during the summer months to prevent overheating and add a few during the cold winter months to keep the internal fires burning.

In China, people often serve food on traditional red lacquer dishes. I have read that the warmth-generating color transmits warming energies to your body with each bite you take. While I am not certain that investing in a set of these plates will ensure smooth skin and a happy Heart, I do know that being mindful of what you put on those plates will definitely help. Be sure to eat such Heart-healthy foods as chard, endive, watercress, artichokes, asparagus, grapefruit, rhubarb, beets, tomatoes, radishes, and red peppers year-round. Also remember that cooked foods are better than raw foods in this instance.

In the summer months when your Heart needs a little extra care, be sure to add some more bitter foods to the mix too. As mentioned earlier, wild cucumber, celery, and dark leafy greens such as arugula, kale, and spinach are all examples of helpful bitter foods, as are vinegar, saffron, and turmeric.

Be in bed before 11:00 P.M. and try to nap or meditate briefly each day between 11:00 A.M. and 1:00 P.M. That is when your Qi replenishes your Heart.

Wash your face with green tea to eliminate wrinkles and reduce the black circles under your eyes. Green tea helps disperse Heat and Dampness, contains rich antioxidant catechins, and can powerfully clear your body of free radicals.

When visiting your Chinese medicine practitioner, ask if any of the following natural herbs can help you, or look for some of the following ingredients in the beauty products you currently use or are shopping for.

- *Bai zhi* (root of *Angelica dahurica*)

  The root of this plant is used to inhibit the growth of bacteria, reduce inflammation from infection, and improve the skin's blood circulation. It generally makes your skin feel silky, soft, and dewy.

- *Bai ji* (root of *Bletilla striata*)

  When used medicinally, this root helps stop bleeding and speeds the recovery of wounds. It is known to reduce facial scars and spots, as well as to heal acne. It is also used to make skin smooth and shiny.

- *Bai guo* (semen *Ginkgo*)

  This ointment effectively inhibits the spread of fungus on the skin and energetically supports the Lung and the Kidney Meridians, which oxygenate the blood and play a big part in nurturing the skin. When used topically, it helps eliminate acne and rosacea.

- *Bai fuling* (*Smilax china*)

  Recommended to strengthen Spleen energy, this herb reduces water retention and calms the mind. It also improves circulation and immune functionality. It can help minimize acne, skin spots, and wrinkles.

- *Bai jili* (*Fructus tribuli*)

  When taken internally, this herb sedates the Liver *Yang* energy, supports Kidney *Yin* energy, helps vision, and heals wounds. It has antioxidant properties, enhances testosterone production, and improves fertility in both men and women. It also makes skin soft and supple.

- *Bai suzi* (*Perilla frutescens*)

  If you are looking for something to help minimize yellow age spots and wrinkles, this herb may be your answer. It also helps reduce asthma, coughing, and constipation.

Wear fabrics that breathe so your skin doesn't let too much perspiration—and the Heart *Qi* carried with it—escape.

Add soft pinks and blushes to your wardrobe throughout the summer to help some of the Heat energy that is lost through sweat return to your body. During the rest of the year, wear bold, daring ruby reds and scarlets to help replenish Heart *Qi* after an intense physical workout.

Arrange and display a large bouquet of red flowers where you are sure to see and enjoy them in your home or office. It doesn't have to cost you much— wild roses grow rampant in the summer so clip a few from the garden or roadside and enjoy their aroma as well as their energy. Bringing amaryllis and poinsettias indoors during the winter will also bring warm energy into your home and Heart!

Listen to meditative music or hum the so tone of the pentatonic scale on your way to work today.

Engage in craft projects, sculpt, paint, weave, play an instrument, sing, or act. Creativity energizes the Heart and shows in both your work and your face.

Watch a comedy and laugh loud, long, and *heartily*! Laughter not only brings healthful energy to the surface of your skin, it supports muscles too, giving your face more tone and definition.

Enjoy the scents of chamomile, frankincense, lavender, sandalwood, or ylang-ylang. They are great for your *Shen*, which is housed in the Heart and which also adds radiance to your overall countenance.

Meditate freely and often. Your skin will look relaxed and supple when all of your tension has been released.

Clench and open your fist several times in succession. Be especially sure that your middle finger is held tightly against the center of your palm when squeezing, as this will invigorate the flow of energy and blood along the Heart Meridian and add luminance to your face.

Massage acupuncture points along the Heart Meridian below the elbow and the Small Intestine Meridian in the hands for the same reason (see illustrations on page 95).

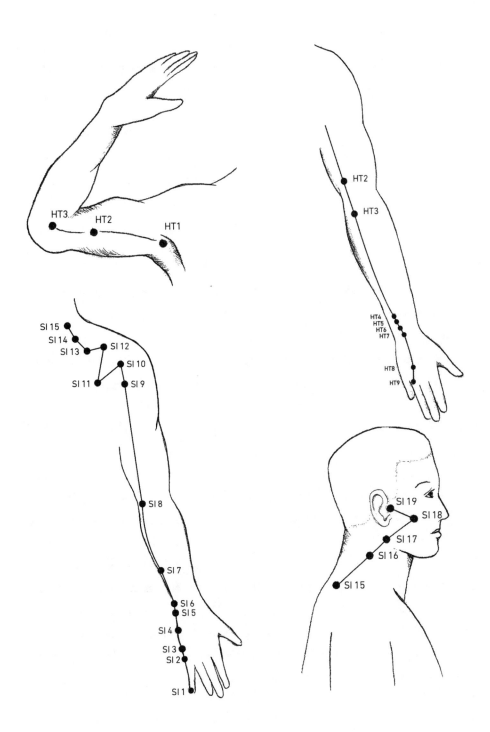

HT3
HT2
HT1

HT2
HT3

SI 15
SI 14
SI 13
SI 12
SI 10
SI 11
SI 9

HT4
HT5
HT6
HT7
HT8
HT9

SI 8

SI 19
SI 18
SI 17
SI 16
SI 15

SI 7

SI 6
SI 5
SI 4
SI 3
SI 2

SI 1

Since key acupuncture points regulating your Heart run from your armpit to the tip of your pinky finger, extend your arms and rotate them, making small circular motions to help jumpstart blood and Qi circulation.

Follow Norma's lead and seek cosmetic acupuncture from a qualified practitioner. It will not only clear your complexion, it will improve your energy, digestion, and the quality of your sleep as well. By using points on your body to stimulate your face, and points on your face to stimulate your body, this acupuncture treatment creates complete energetic balance inside and out.

PATIENT-TESTED TRUTHS

Twenty-five-year-old Joie came to me because she was frustrated that she still had trouble with acne. When she was a teenager, she understood that it was a normal part of her development, but having to contend with it when she was in her midtwenties and trying to put her best face forward in the working world was tough. Although her job was high pressure at times, she was happy that she was meeting lots of new people and that her flexible schedule allowed her to work out during lunchtime at a nearby gym. But while exercise helped her derail her stress, it didn't completely eliminate it. She felt the need to constantly perform at her best to meet her quota as a salesperson and to meet the expectations of her new boss, who was a highly critical but knowledgeable person. Upon Joie's first visit, it was clear that she was experiencing stagnated Liver Qi, which causes internal heat and digestive problems, as well as Dampness. Losing fluid during excessive exercise compounded the problem by generating even more heat in the body. The Liver Qi stagnation as well as Dampness and Heat in the internal organs manifested as diarrhea and menstrual cramps in addition to acne. A course of acupuncture treatment and customized herbal remedies to disperse the stagnated Qi, and to clear the Dampness and Heat has significantly reduced Joie's symptoms. Healthier coping skills were also discussed to better handle her stress.

A QUICK WORD ABOUT ACNE

Joie's story reminds me to address those of you who, like her, are still experiencing acne well past the time you expected to, or who may have adolescent children who are struggling with harsh blemishes and frequent breakouts. You should note that just as sweat and hormonal changes affect the health of your facial skin, the well-being of several internal organs, including the Heart and Small Intestine, can greatly impact the quality of your skin, too. Because the aim of this book is to provide the basic principles of Chinese medicine as they relate to health, beauty, and vitality, we have only touched upon the first level of relationships that exist between internal and external organs. However, traditional Chinese medicine understands the body to be far more layered than I have described so far. Many, many more connections exist between certain body parts and the five primary organs and their partner organs. When viewed in their entirety, these connections illustrate just how much of an amazing circuit board of energy the human body really is. For now, let me dig down at least one more layer to show you the relationship between the different parts of your face and the organs that also impact their health. These relationships exist in addition to the primary relationship the skin has with the Heart.

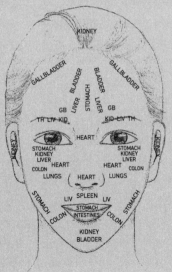

The illustration on page 97 summarizes the association between each acne-prone area of your face and the organ that directly impacts that area. As always, nurture those associated organs and you will greatly improve the color, texture, and elasticity of your skin.

To rid yourself of lingering breakouts or to help that teenager in your life who is dealing with acne, you might want to read the tips in the next section. Although a few of these suggestions may sound familiar, as you've read variations of them in earlier parts of this book, we realize that most of the teens you share this information with are likely to be encountering it for the first time. We have tried to make the presentation of material accessible at a glance. However, if they have the time and inclination to read the whole book, please encourage them to do so. They are at the perfect age to begin the kind of whole-body care that will keep them healthy, youthful, and beautiful for their entire lives!

PIMPLES MADE SIMPLE
A Guide to Eradicating Acne in Your Lifetime!

Breakouts on the upper forehead extending from each brow to the center of your scalp line may indicate a need for extra care to the Urinary Bladder. In that case, try to let go of your fears and anxieties. I understand juggling work, family, and community obligations is tough for many adults, and social pressures, grades, homework, and more add to the day-to-day stress of the typical teen, but breathe deeply, meditate, and focus on what is positive in your life. Watch your intake of salt, wear your favorite black suit or t-shirt to help fortify your *Jing*, splash your face with water on breaks or in between classes if you must, and take relaxing baths or long showers in the evenings. Most of all, recognize that this crazy phase in your life will pass and that you will learn to balance all that comes your way in time and with practice.

Breakouts on the ears may indicate a need for extra care to the Kidneys. Be sure to follow all of the advice offered previously for the care of your

Urinary Bladder (the Kidneys' partner). I'd also suggest drinking enough water and exercising in the late afternoon between 3:00 and 5:00 P.M.

Breakouts on your cheeks to the right or left of your nostrils may indicate a need for extra care to your Lungs. Let go of any feelings of loss or rejection you may be holding on to, especially if you've recently broken up with a loved one or if the dynamics at work, home, school, or with your friends are a little tense right now. Take a walk and breathe in the fresh air. Wear an article of white clothing and a piece of jewelry made from a precious metal such as sterling silver. Are you eating more garlic or onions than usual? Or not enough? Think about that when ordering your next pizza as the Lungs and their partner organ, the Large Intestine, are both sensitive and responsive to pungent foods! Eating just the right amount helps. Also be sure to check for allergies... and don't smoke!

Breakouts on the nose may indicate a need for extra care to the Heart. Play music that makes you happy, and dance around your home whether you feel like it or not. In just a few minutes you will have sent your blues away. Don't sweat the small stuff. Wear a red scarf, red tie, or bold red sneakers. Get creative by decorating a favorite room at home or your locker to reflect more of your true self. Speak up about how you feel on any topic of importance to you, whether it relates to the world at large or your world at home. Laugh more often—not at others—but at funny movies and jokes. Eat bitter foods in the midst of a breakout—having an arugula salad or kale chips at lunch can help. Put a little sandalwood or ylang-ylang essential oil on your wrists. The smell won't be the only thing pleasing to your nose—its power to clear pimples will be too!

Breakouts just above the furrow of your brows or on your brows may indicate a need for extra care to the Liver. Let go of any residual anger you may have. If you've lost an account or a baseball game, or if you didn't do as well in your performance review or on your math test as you wanted to, don't berate yourself (or even your boss or teacher under your breath). Vow to do better next time and move on. Exercise good judgment. Wear lucky socks in the perfect shade of blue and green. Add plants to your environment—and remember to care for them too, because they'll be caring for you! Also try to add more sour foods to your diet if you have not been doing so—and I don't mean Sour Patch candy. That qualifies as *sweet* more than *sour*! Try a lemon, grapefruit, or some other citrus fruit that makes you pucker. Give yourself a night off to stay home and listen to some mellow music or to curl up in bed with a good book.

Breakouts in the groove above your upper lip may indicate a need for extra care to the Spleen. Try to let go of your cares and worries and remember to nurture the kid in you no matter what your age. Play a little every now and then! Curb your intake of sugars—especially refined sugars—if you are eating them in excess. Enjoy naturally sweet foods such as fresh or dried fruits instead. And stay away from greasy fast foods! Wear the color yellow for a quick pick-me-up and a fabric blend that wicks sweat away from your body. Be sure to launder work-out clothes regularly; let your shower towel dry fully before putting it in the hamper where it will get musty; change out of damp and sweaty clothes quickly and clean up after spills in your home as soon as they happen. Use a dehumidifier in your bedroom if it is particularly damp. All these steps will not only improve your complexion, they'll provide a boost to your thought and reasoning abilities too. Always a plus when you've got a big meeting coming up or around finals time!

Breakouts on the upper lip may indicate a need for extra care to the Stomach. The same advice just offered for the Spleen holds true here too. (The Stomach is the Spleen's partner.) Also, don't be shy about singing along to your favorite music. I'm serious—it will align the lips with the organs, thoughts, and emotions that nurture them best.

Breakouts on the lower chin may indicate a need for extra care to the Kidneys, Urinary Bladder, and reproductive system. Do everything recommended earlier for the Kidneys and Urinary Bladder and also be sure to add one or more of the following to your diet, especially in the winter: eggplant, black figs, black mushrooms, black sesame seeds, black beans, and dark walnuts. Lastly, get enough rest. I know that client dinners and the need for just a little "me" time when the rest of the family is asleep keeps adults up until all hours of the night, and that homework and extracurricular activities keep teens awake too. The hours after 11:00 P.M. are sometimes the only free ones you have to read or watch TV, but being in bed—and actually falling asleep—before then is crucial to your health, beauty, willpower, motivation, and coordination, now and in the future too!

MY SECRET TO AN AGELESS COMPLEXION

If it is true that we are what we eat, then eating congee will make you beautiful and healthy. The following is a recipe I suggest to my patients who are hoping to improve the overall health of their skin. This congee involves millet, a grain that is particularly healthy for your Heart, Small Intestine, and, you guessed it, your complexion.

Recipe for Complexion-Enhancing Congee
(MAKES 4 SERVINGS)

INGREDIENTS:

1 cup of foxtail millet

5 cups of water

¼ cup of lotus seeds

¼ cup of Lilium (dried daylilies, which you can purchase online or at your local Chinese food mart)

10 pieces of red dates (jujubes)

Rinse the millet before adding it to a pot with the 5 cups of water. Bring to a boil over medium heat, then reduce the heat to a simmer and cover.

When the millet is 70 percent cooked and the remaining water is still rich and creamy, add the seeds and *Lilium* and stir for two to three minutes.

Ladle into serving bowls and top with the red dates.

Serve warm for breakfast or as a nourishing late-day snack.

Norma's Musings on the Art of Putting Your Best Face Forward

Many times, when people wear a lot of makeup, it looks as if they are wearing a mask. Unfortunately, I associate heavy makeup with corpses too. But if you look at the face of someone who is working out or has just taken a brisk walk, they look positively glowing. Their skin is all dewy and energized. They are flush with color. Skin without makeup is beautiful. Sweaty skin is especially beautiful. The color of skin after exercise is like nothing else. Because the blood is flowing, there is movement and grace to it. Having healthy skin has to do with being alive. Stripping off the mask and letting the skin underneath it breathe is one way to have a radiant complexion. Eating a healthy diet is another. Moving about, and of course, getting rest to balance all that activity is imperative. Acupuncture, as I mentioned before, amps up the quality of your sleep, so I find it invaluable to achieving beautiful skin. There is no product in the world that will give you the same enlivened look that acupuncture does. Using olive oil soap in the shower and refreshing throughout the day with some olive oil liniment combined with calcium helps too. I apply it daily to my face, arms, and legs. And I never wear foundation. I prefer to use a plant-based tanner once or twice a week instead. I find it gives me a light, even tone without ever hiding my complexion. I always think, *If I am hiding my skin under makeup, I'm giving it a reason to be flawed.* Right? It becomes a self-fulfilling prophecy that I'll have bad skin. So I really believe in letting your skin shine naturally. Try it. Take the challenge. It's an incredibly liberating feeling.

7

Seeing Is Believing

SECRETS TO HEALTHY AND BEAUTIFUL EYES

People of all ages are concerned with avoiding fine lines, hooded eyelids, saggy brows, puffiness, and dark circles under their eyes, and of course preventing worsening eyesight and conditions such as dry eye or glaucoma as they get older. **Dr. Yang, what can you tell readers to guide them toward better care of their eyes?**

It's obvious that the eyes are very important organs. They are supported mostly by the Liver and the Gallbladder, so when either of these two organs suffers, the eyes reflect their pain and suffering. For example, seeing black spots or experiencing blurred vision, vertigo, or dizzy spells all result from the compromised health of the Liver or Gallbladder. The root cause of migraines or headaches that begin in the temporal area behind the eyes can also be traced to an imbalance of energies in these organs. So can jaundice—the yellow discoloration of the eyes when a diseased liver fails to discard bilirubin from the body as it is supposed to. Other diseases of the liver, including hepatitis or cirrhosis, can also pose threats to the health and appearance of your eyes. Practitioners of Chinese medicine can look at your eyes and tell a lot from whether they are dull or focused and spirited.

Given the profound connection these organs have with our eyes, it is deeply disturbing to see how modern medicine continues to remove the Gallbladder as a defense against chronic gallstones without first treating the Liver and endocrine system with various integrative medical practices. The potential repercussions for the eyes can be very serious.

The way to care for the eyes is to nurture the Liver and Gallbladder with every tool at your disposal. **But before we list those tools, we really should talk about the eyes' wondrous and unique connection with every other part of the body.** Did you know that puffy lids let us know something is going on with the Spleen? That red, bloodshot, or irritated eyes hint that the Heart may need some nurturing too? Or that sties are an indication that there is too much Damp Heat in your system?

It is said that the eyes are the windows to the soul, but this saying is more than just a metaphor. Because they connect with each of the primary and partner organs, and these organs connect with our mental, emotional, and spiritual qualities, the eyes actually do provide a glimpse of the whole health of our being. Although the Liver and Gallbladder are the primary and partner organs governing the eyes, the more specific feature pairings are as follows:

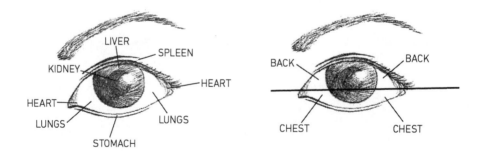

- The cornea and iris correspond with the Liver.
- The arteries and veins correspond with the Heart.
- The top eyelid corresponds with the Spleen; the bottom eyelid corresponds with the Spleen's partner, the Stomach.

- The white of your eyes, called the sclera, corresponds with the Lungs.
- The lens of the eye and the pupil correspond with the Kidneys.

As a result, caring for your eyes also means caring for each of the organs just discussed in all the ways we talk about throughout this book. It also means being especially careful about exposure to certain external pathogens as we age and our immune system slows down. Some things to guard against include:

- **Exposure to excessive Heat energy,** which can cause swelling, redness, teariness, pain, and bleeding.
- **Exposure to excessive Cold energy,** which can cause blurred vision, pain, supersensitivity to light, and teariness.
- **Exposure to extreme Wind energy,** which can result in twitching, pressure, or pain in the eyes and around the eye orbits, general redness and inflammation of the eyelids, sensitivity to light, teariness, and temporary paralysis of the eye and the eyelid's movement as in cases of Bell's palsy.
- **Exposure to excessive Dry energy,** which can cause redness, itching, burning, and dryness.
- **Exposure to excessive Damp energy,** which can cause swelling of the eyelids, jaundice, blurred and/or double vision, pain, and the buildup of mucus in the eyes.

You should also guard against energy stagnation as this can lead to headaches, eye pain, congested veins, and the formation of tumors. Be sure to get up and move around as frequently as possible when doing work that involves your eyes for long periods of time.

A FEW EASY STEPS YOU CAN TAKE TO HELP NURTURE YOUR EYES

Again, find a way to deal constructively with feelings of anger, resentment, bitterness, irritation, and general discontent. When left unchecked, these emotions attack the Liver and Gallbladder and ultimately disrupt your vision too. They affect your physical eyes *and* they negatively color the way you perceive and experience the world around you.

Cut back on alcohol and coffee. Both are known to cause excessive Dampness in your Blood Qi, stopping the healthy flow of nutrients to your eyes. It is recommended that you drink green tea instead.

Add sour foods such as lemons, kiwi, green olives, and green grapes to your mealtime menu in the spring. These foods help restore the body's fluids when they're needed, keeping your eyes moist, clear, and sharp.

Eat more cooked green leafy vegetables, including kale, spinach, collard greens, and chard.

Open your eyes to the healing powers of cyan. Wearing an accessory in this powerful blend of blue and green is bound to make a grand visual statement—one that positively impacts your eyesight and the visual impression you make on others too.

Spread blues and greens liberally around your home and office in the form of plant life, textiles, and art, especially during the springtime when the Liver and Gallbladder, and consequently the eyes, are most vulnerable.

Wear sunglasses to protect your eyes from pathogens carried by the wind.

Be sure to get your beauty rest between the hours of 11:00 P.M. and 3:00 A.M. This is when your Qi is doing its nightly repair work on your Liver.

To aid your sleep and to ensure that your eyes are especially well rejuvenated, wear an eye mask to bed—preferably one in soothing shades of blue and green.

Warm up for the day ahead of you by singing the mi tone of the pentatonic scale to yourself and holding that note as long as you can.

Enjoy wearing a bold piece of handcrafted wooden jewelry. Remember that wood's organic energy fortifies your Liver so it also supports your eyes. If you are always so busy you "can't see the forest for the trees," wearing wooden jewelry will help you feel and experience the mutually healing relationship we are meant to have with nature.

Practice compassion and forgiveness. It can help you see the other side of an argument more clearly and bring about harmony between your Liver and your eyes, your mind and your body, and yourself and the larger world around you.

Massage your Liver 3 and Gallbladder 37 points per the following illustrations. This will enable everything along your Liver Meridian to function optimally. Try it and see. Literally!

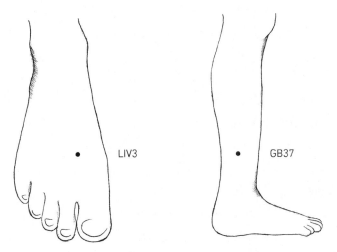

PATIENT-TESTED TRUTHS

Forty-five-year-old Elena woke up one day and panicked because she couldn't read the emails she always checks first thing in the morning. No matter how large she made the type, it still appeared blurry. She's a book editor who looks at text all day long, so she really needs to keep her eyes sharp. How could a change like this happen overnight?

Her eye doctor said that age had caught up with her when she wasn't looking. Her sight had been worsening for quite some time, but she wasn't paying much attention until her eyes sent out an S.O.S. He prescribed reading glasses, and rather than telling her to accept worsening eyesight as a matter of aging, he also suggested that she slow down a little more and take time to notice whatever else her body might be telling her.

Elena followed the doctor's advice and came to see me as a proactive measure. I gave her what I like to call a general *health lift,* with an extra emphasis on improving her vision. In addition to the acupuncture treatments I administered, I taught her a few simple acupressure techniques she could continue to use at home. After her next annual eye exam, she reported that her eyes were doing well. When asked about her general health, she said she had never felt better. A few weeks after her treatment she noticed that she was able to walk longer distances and move about more freely. Long gone was the pain from plantar fasciitis—a condition that causes the tendons in the arches of the feet to hurt. I asked if she was still doing the acupressure techniques I showed her and she said, "Every day!" Her commitment and perseverance clearly helped her repair some of the faults along the Liver Meridian that she wasn't aware of until her need for glasses opened her eyes to them. See the next illustration for the location of key acupressure points around your eyes that you can work on too to improve your eyesight, tendons and ligaments, nails, digestion, sleep, and so much more. Rub the points softly for a few minutes before going to bed each night and you will awaken to better health in the morning. It never ceases to amaze my patients how treating one organ along the meridian can improve the health of all the others in its path.

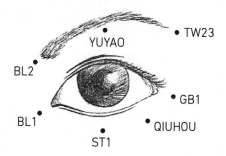

MY SECRET TO MAINTAINING THAT SPARKLE IN YOUR EYES

The following is another favorite recipe I suggest to my patients. This one is to help improve the overall health of their eyes. Try it. You will not only feel the difference, you will see it too.

Congee Recipe for Bright Eyes
(MAKES 4 SERVINGS)

INGREDIENTS:

½ cup of rice

4 cups of water

½ cup of goji berries

¼ cup of almonds and/or hazelnuts

Wash rice thoroughly. Put the rice and the water in a pot and bring to a boil over medium heat. Reduce heat to a simmer and cover.

Reserve a few nuts for toppings, and then grind the rest into a powder.

When the rice is 70 percent cooked and the remaining water is still rich and creamy, add the powder and goji berries.

Stir for two to three minutes.

Serve hot with the reserved nuts as garnish.

For an equally tasty variation on this recipe replace the goji berries with muddled mulberries. Both are excellent for your eyes!

Norma's Musings on the Windows to the Soul

When you are talking to someone—I mean really talking to them—you look in their eyes. For me, the eyes are the most expressive feature of the face. We can tell what people are thinking when we look in their eyes. I can see how you are reacting to me. If you're affected by something emotionally, your eyes may get teary. They may become more animated. Your eyes can't hide their response. They just don't lie. If we are observant enough, we can really get to know each other through our eyes. They infuse an emotional energy into the entire face. How we wrap our eyes with makeup or how we frame them with glasses also says something about us. The eyes are a form of expression and communication even when nothing else is being said.

I tend to do very little to my eyes. I let them speak for themselves. I wear a little bit of natural mascara produced by RMS; I use my olive oil liniment as moisturizer; and I wear glasses. My glasses are as much of a statement as makeup in revealing who I am.

The most challenging restoration of tired eyes is to simply close them. Especially because we look at so many digital screens these days, it is helpful to give your eyes a rest throughout the day. When they are open, they are just too busy. Great times to take rest periods are during meals and while you are on the phone. I will also use a salt or lavender mask to help relax my eyes.

Looking your best in this case has a double meaning. You want to preserve the way your eyes look at the world around you as much as you want the world around you to look and see something interesting in your eyes. Maintaining the beauty of your eyes definitely means maintaining their health and the heath of the organs that support them.

8

Giving Chinese Medicine
a Fair Hearing

HOW HAVING HEALTHY EARS IS GOOD FOR YOUR WHOLE BEING

I'm not sure what kind of beauty advice you could possibly give us regarding our ears as most of our daily regimens address them minimally, except, of course, to keep them clean. **But Dr. Yang, you always have something interesting to tell us, so I have to ask, what can we do to improve the health and well-being of our ears?**

I'm so glad you raised this topic. Chinese medicine tells us that the ears are among our most important features! More than 200 acupuncture points connect them to other parts of the body. While the untrained eye cannot identify all of these points, the unique shape of our ears provides some basic clues as to which parts correspond to which primary internal organs. If you look closely at your ear in the mirror, you will notice that it looks like an upside-down fetus as it lies in its mother's womb. (That alone makes one's ears beautiful to me!) The head of the fetus rests at the ear's base, where the lobe is. The recessed area near the ear canal represents the baby's chest, while the outer ridge, called the helix, corresponds to its spine. And tucked just inside of that ridge is where the baby's arms, hands, and feet rest. Look at the following illustration to see what I mean.

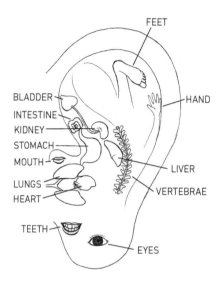

Applying acupuncture needles to certain points on the ear can help stimulate the energy in these other areas of the body. So too can applying acupressure. For instance, gently massaging the lobes can help relieve headaches, tooth pain, and eyestrain, and can also bring a healthy glow to your cheeks. Gently massaging the notch nearest to the entrance of the ear canal can improve your blood flow. Rubbing the region just above that improves digestion, while massaging along the inside of the ridge running parallel to the helix, known as the anti-helix, can help reduce stress or discomfort in your back, shoulders, and neck, and so forth.

It is generally suggested that you massage these points twenty times each to avoid under- or overstimulating them. You should do this twice a day.

Energetically, the ears connect with the Heart, Lungs, Kidneys, Liver, and Spleen. Consequently, energetic abnormalities within any of these organs will be reflected on the ears' surface. For example, growths such as sebaceous cysts appearing on the ears indicate a possible *Qi* and Blood Stagnation in the organ corresponding to that spot on the ear. Redness indicates the presence of excessive Heat and inflammation, while eczema indicates the presence of Damp Heat in the organ associated with that area.

Interestingly enough, even modern medicine is catching on to the connection between the ears and the health of certain other organs. More than thirty reputable studies—including one from the widely respected Mayo Clinic—suggest that the presence of a diagonal earlobe crease may indicate the presence of coronary artery disease for men under the age of sixty.

The ears really are great diagnostic tools. It seems as if they not only listen, they have a lot to say too. Heeding their message will not only keep them free of marks and blemishes, it will also help you address larger underlying issues that could be impacting your overall health and beauty.

EASY THINGS YOU CAN DO TO NURTURE YOUR EARS

Because the ears and the function of hearing correlate with the Kidneys and Urinary Bladder, everything I previously suggested that you do to nurture these organs applies to the ears as well. So if you have any of the symptoms mentioned earlier, are experiencing tinnitus, finding it hard to hear what those around you are saying, or you are suffering from frequent earaches, be sure to seek medical help and also support your medical practitioner's efforts by doing all that you can to nourish your Kidneys. This includes suiting up in all black clothing, eating more black-colored foods to increase the *Postnatal Jing* that supports hearing, and watching your salt intake as it can make you retain Dampness in your ears. Also be sure to:

Pull your collar up high or wear earmuffs, a hat, headband, or scarf to protect your ears from the various pathogens introduced to the body in Cold and/or Windy weather.

Wear noise-canceling earplugs or headphones when there is construction going on around you or if you must use loud equipment for work.

Enjoy some quiet time. Overstimulation of the sensitive ears can also overstimulate the other parts of the body they are connected to, generating both excessive Heat and anxiety. Allow your ears to rest a little each day.

Even if you have no such ailments, but you wish to give your overall health a boost, massage both ears in the morning to provide your organs with an extra push to get you through the day and again in the evening to help those same organs relax and recharge.

Massage the soles of your feet. The Kidney Meridian actually begins at the bottoms of the feet, so rubbing them or even stamping them will help get their energies moving, aiding all the organs in their path, including the ears.

Pursue acupressure and acupuncture treatments on the ears. Both are powerful therapies for reducing pain in various parts of the body and eliminating cravings for substances that are unhealthy for you, such as sweets and tobacco.

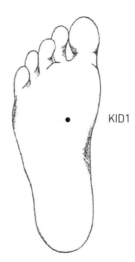

KID1

PATIENT-TESTED TRUTHS

Fifty-two-year-old Julie had recently begun to experience tinnitus. She came to me hoping that I could help. When evaluating her overall health, I learned that she had been treated for diabetes most of her adult life. She didn't make the connection between the two conditions until she consulted with me. From a Chinese medicine perspective, the Kidneys store and provide *Yin* energy to the entire body. Diabetes develops when one's *Yin Qi,* or cooling energy, is deficient. As a result, many of the other organs along the same meridian begin suffering, too, including the ears, which was exactly what was happening to Julie. The *Qi* intended to support her hearing was so deficient by the time it reached her ears that it caused the tinnitus. Julie ultimately responded well to acupuncture and to treatment with a special rehmannia root formula. Although many patients still take insulin, the aim of Chinese medicine in treating diabetes with such herbs is to help restore the balance of energy to the point where the body can regulate its glucose level on its own. With continued visits Julie is now managing her diabetes more effectively. And the ringing in her ears has stopped completely. While she is happy about the peace and quiet she is experiencing again, she is grateful that the ringing served as a warning bell for her to monitor her diabetes more closely.

A WORD ABOUT EAR PIERCINGS . . . AND OTHER BODY PIERCINGS

Before we move on from the topic of ears, I'd like to address the growing trend of multiple piercings, not only on the ears but on other parts of the body, too. While acupuncturists stimulate specific points on the ear with fine needles in the treatment of a wide variety of conditions, we are always aware of the effect each needle will have on the point we're invigorating and its corresponding organ. That is not necessarily true of the employee at the jewelry store or body-art shop where most people go to get their ears, tongue, navel, and other parts of their anatomy pierced. If you are thinking about getting one or more new piercings, it's important that you consider the possible impact on your *Qi* and overall health before doing so.

Because the jewelry worn in these piercings is often made of metals, and metals are conductors of energy, it has the potential to interfere with the flow of your body's *Qi,* especially when this metal is in place for hours, days, weeks, or months on end. In the short term, a stimulated acupuncture point can energize you. But the long-term stimulation from a body piercing can have a very different effect, impacting and potentially challenging the specific organs associated with the pierced region.

If you do already have multiple body piercings, it is suggested that you remove your jewelry at night to let your body rest from the sustained invigoration of acupuncture points, Also consider wearing jewelry made from inert materials such as wood or porcelain instead.

Norma's Musings on Ear Care and the Sound of Silence

When I was twelve years old I went with several girls from my neighborhood to Italian Harlem to get our ears pierced. I wore lots of different kinds of earrings then, but today I have a minimalist approach to jewelry and don't wear earrings at all. Even if I did, I think I'd shy away from the trend to have multiple piercings because of my love of change. I'd be reluctant to do anything so permanent. Whenever I contemplate making any long-lasting change to my appearance I always think, *What if I hate it later?* There is a belief that every seven years we transform, evolve, and grow as individuals, naturally entering into a new stage of life and development. If this is truly the case, our perspective and tastes will no doubt change with each phase, too. Today the nicest thing I do for my ears is take some time to indulge them in complete silence. There is music playing in the store all day—beautiful music—but it can be distracting when you are working. And all the sounds on the city streets when you are getting around town can be overstimulating too. Because of that, I find sitting in total quiet to be a complete luxury that is good not only for your ears, but for all of the other organs in your body too. If you don't already do it now, take a moment of silence at the start and end to each day. It's really very gratifying.

9

Common Scents Advice

SECRETS TO HAVING A HEALTHY AND BEAUTIFUL NOSE

When I was growing up in a predominantly Irish neighborhood, it seemed everyone around me had pretty, little, turned-up noses, and I remember feeling that because of the size and shape of my nose I didn't fit that particular definition of pretty. I know some people who, even as adults, are concerned about the size and shape of their nose. Today I appreciate mine and all other types—flat noses, round noses, long noses, and aquiline noses—as much as I do petite noses. They all have character, but since they serve a central role in our well-being and occupy a central spot on our faces, too, I particularly like healthy noses. No one wants to be around or have a stuffed or runny nose. As we've learned from you already, Dr. Yang, every external feature has unexpected relationships with internal organs that really do impact our overall health and appearance. **So what can you tell us about the role of our nose in maintaining health and beauty?**

In Chinese medicine, the Lungs are the primary organs associated with the nose. But, just as some of the other facial features we've discussed so far let us know when something is amiss with another organ in the body, the nose provides similar clues about possible energy imbalances. For instance, widespread redness on the entire nose indicates excessive Heat in the Lungs. Redness concentrated on the upper third and the bridge of the nose may indicate excessive Heat in your Heart. If your nose is dark blue or marked by broken capillaries it may mean that your Liver energy is too stagnated. Also, when nose hairs turn gray, it is a sign of Kidney Deficiency. A frequent bloody nose means your surroundings are too dry. The vast majority of people with a horizontal crease in the bridge of their nose tend to have Stomach and digestive problems including pain, indigestion, diarrhea, or constipation. If, in addition to these other signs, your nose is also sweaty, you should have your blood pressure checked. And most commonly, a runny nose with clear discharge can indicate Wind Cold Qi in the Lungs while a thick yellowish discharge from the nose indicates Wind Heat Qi invasion.

The nose is one of the most prominent features of the face. Ensuring its health means ensuring the healthy image you put forward to the world. In the animal kingdom, signs of health are what attract potential mates. The same is true with humans, so don't take the allure of a clear, healthy nose for granted.

But let's get back to the many ways the nose works in conjunction with the Lungs. The nose's sense of smell is a prime example of how the two work together. Smell helps you determine what may or may not be healthy to inhale. This is why this sense is so strong in women during pregnancy. It warns them of toxins and impurities in the air and also signals them to keep away from spoiled foods, both of which can introduce harmful pathogens into the body and potentially harm both mother and baby. But while the healthy functioning of the nose is expected to help the Lungs remain free and clear of airborne germs and dangers, the Lungs are expected to help the nose, too. If your nose is congested due to a common cold, allergies, or a sinus infection, your Lung energy may be the problem. Instead of reaching for antihistamines, what you really should do is try to take better care of your Lungs so they can support your nasal passages. Borrowing from the many things we've already discussed about how to nurture your Lungs and adding a few more tips, here is what you can do to keep your Lungs, and subsequently your nose, in optimal health:

Let go of the people, memories, and situations that make you feel sad. The Lungs are actually tissue-paper-thin so they can inflate and deflate with ease, but when the Lungs absorb the weight of your emotions, they become too heavy to do their job well. Did you know that when you sigh, it is often a sign that your Lungs are trying to rid themselves of excess emotion?

Remain sleeping until after 5:00 A.M. each day. The hours between 3:00 and 5:00 A.M. are when the Lungs are being repaired. Pull the bed covers over you tightly so you can keep warm throughout the night. This will help you sleep more soundly and guard against anything waking you before you're ready.

Pay attention to what you eat. Do you eat enough pungent foods? The first examples that come to mind are onions, endive, and cauliflower, but I forgot earlier to mention another favorite—mint! Whatever pungent foods you eat, strive to enjoy them in moderation.

Wear white clothes, especially around the throat and chest area, and during the crisp fall weather. White brings clear energy to the Lungs, which in turn, enables the nose to breathe freely.

Massage your Lung 9 acupuncture point—and while you're at it, also massage your nose to help improve the circulation of energy.

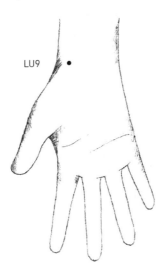

LU9

Check your home and office for any irritants that may be lurking there, including chemicals in your laundry detergent and household cleaning products, as well as hair sprays and deodorants. Also be sure to check that your air-conditioning filters and heating ducts are clean.

If your radiators emit too much Dry Heat, be sure to use a humidifier to help moisten the air, too.

To help deal with frequent nosebleeds, cut back on foods and beverages with high Heat energy, including spicy foods and sauces like Sriracha, alcohol, coffee, tea, and even rich chocolates as the additional Heat energy may be contributing to the problem. Also avoid over-the-counter cold and flu medicines and other drugs that are known to thin the blood.

Lastly, be attentive to how you smell. If you notice a rank or fishy odor anywhere on your body, this can mean that an imbalance of *Qi* in your Lungs or Large Intestine needs to be addressed. (Some of the other odors that suggest *Qi* imbalances according to Chinese medicine are as follows: a rancid or foul smell correlates to potential imbalances in the Liver and Gallbladder; a burnt smell correlates to potential imbalances in the Heart and Small Intestine; a sweet or fragrant smell correlates to potential imbalances in the Spleen and Stomach; and a putrid or rotting smell correlates to potential imbalances in the Kidneys and Urinary Bladder. These odors can mean different things depending upon whether they occur in just one area or are pervasive throughout the body, so check in with your Chinese medicine practitioner if you detect any of them. One of these organs may need some extra attention.)

PATIENT-TESTED TRUTHS

Fifty-six-year-old Zoe came to me complaining that she was sick for most of the month of September. She said she had a lingering cold that began with a bad sore throat. She just wanted to feel better, look in the mirror again, and see that her red nose and tired puffy eyes had returned to normal. She had breast cancer a few years back and was in total remission, but her internal *Qi* was weak as a result. This made her susceptible to multiple external pathogens. Her initial sore throat, which was accompanied by a fever and thick mucus in her nose, was caused by the invasion of Wind Heat *Qi* into the body. Medicating Zoe's symptoms didn't help. Oftentimes, medications—whether prescribed or bought over the counter—will just exacerbate the problem. They tend to dry up the mucus in the nasal passages or temporarily control the infection, but, as Zoe can now tell you, they do not address the *Qi* Deficiency in the Lungs. This leaves the achy, feverish, sore-throat sufferer open to new pathogens when the medication stops. In Zoe's case she ended up with a cold. As the weather changed, coughing, sneezing, and a runny nose with clear discharge ensued due to an invasion of Wind Cold *Qi*. (Some would say this is why it's called a cold!) To finally help Zoe's body rebalance its energies and heal itself, I treated her with acupuncture and a customized herbal remedy based on a classical formula, *Fang Feng Tong Sheng San*. I also showed her key acupressure points on the hand and the back of the head to massage whenever she feels the first signs of either a sore throat or cold coming on.

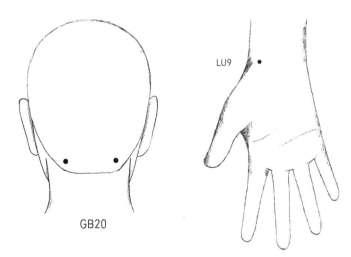

GB20

LU9

Zoe was given weekly acupuncture treatments for a period of six months and has happily been free of problems for the last twelve months. Hopefully these simple tools can help you feel your best while also helping you look your best throughout whatever weather changes each new season brings.

Norma's Musings on the Power of Scent

There is no denying that scent can affect us quite powerfully. Many people enjoy aromatherapy for this reason. If you have any doubts about the nose's link to our emotional core, and the important role it plays in that aspect of our well-being, not just our physical well-being, think about how, after the loss of a loved one, just smelling an article of their clothing can bring back a flood of memories and a very deep connection to their lingering energy. Or how the smells on a return to a childhood home can instantly take you back in time. Think too about pheromones—the sex hormones we emit and their ability to influence the behavior of the opposite sex.

Even fabricated scents can have an incredibly strong pull. I launched a fragrance in 1983 that sold phenomenally well for many years. It was available in two parts—one part was an incense; the other was a beautiful floral that you could layer on top of it. Men could wear it too depending on how much of one you put over the other. I wore it all the time and people would tell me they always knew when I had entered a room. It was an intoxicating scent and I had a cult following for it. People still beg me to bring it back. Now I am partial to plant-based fragrances. I use one at the moment called Restore. It's a scent that lives up to its name. You put it on and you are affected by it. It's an aromatic that also offers immune support. Because it's derived from a plant, you can even drink it as a tea. Wearing it makes you feel a certain way. A scent that can improve your well-being and please the people around you at the same time just feels more fresh and modern to me—more in keeping with the philosophy I have today. As much as I love that people enjoyed the fragrance I previously produced, there are times when you just have to let go of things that aren't necessarily the best for you. If you pay attention to the body's messages as Dr. Yang says, they can guide you to the healthiest choices. In this case, I followed my nose, and my immune system is happy that I did.

10

Smiling Your Way to Radiance

SECRETS TO HEALTHY AND BEAUTIFUL LIPS

Now on to discussing a feature women tend to obsess about almost as much as their hair. We all want our lips to look pleasing, full, and lively. Many of us can recall watching our mothers put on lipstick when we were children. I can still remember the way mine applied hers, gliding the tube along each side of her upper lip and following up with one very sure stroke on the bottom. Then she would snap the cap back on and blot the excess color on a folded tissue, leaving an imprint like a kiss behind. Her lips always looked so beautiful. Wearing lipstick is a rite of passage for women. This was the ritual that made lips look their fullest and boldest before dermal fillers, Botox, and other similar treatments came into vogue. For a long time it was also believed that lipsticks protected the lips from drying and cracking, although that's not always true. **Dr. Yang, what can you tell us about the care and well-being of our lips according to Chinese medicine?**

The lips are very interesting organs. I know women take great care to pick out just the right shade of lip color to wear from the countless options that are newly available every year. I also know how many different procedures and products are available to help make lips look plumper, but there is so much that unadorned, un-adulterated lips can tell us that is crucial to our well-being.

The lips are actually a muscle; therefore, they are supported by and reflect the health of the Spleen and Stomach. Some of the important functions of the Spleen include cleansing bacteria from our blood, boosting our immune system, and containing our blood within its vessels. If you want healthy lips and good health in general, you must care for your Spleen and your Stomach with all the attention you give to the selection of each new season's miracle enhancer, stains, glosses, balms, and liners. The next time you remove your makeup in the evening, look closely at your lips.

- Pale lips indicate a lack of *Qi*, blood, and nutrients. Have you been eating well enough?
- Deep-red, dry lips indicate excess Heat. Is the thermostat in your home or office set too high? Are you properly protecting your lips from the sun when you are outdoors?
- When your lips are cracked, your Spleen and Stomach are telling you they need more fluids to cool them down. Are you drinking enough room-temperature water?
- Too much Heat in the Spleen can cause painful sores to appear on the lips. Are you eating enough cooling or *Yin*-generating foods?
- Bluish-purple lips indicate Blood Stasis. Are you moving around enough? Try to get up from your desk and stretch at different intervals throughout the day. You should also include some form of exercise in your daily routine.
- Sore, chapped, or cut lips can mean you have an infection in your body. Have you been under the weather recently? Are you running a fever?

Taking care of your lips, as with all the other visible features we have discussed, means taking care of the primary and partner organs supporting them. The following tips can help your lips look their best naturally while also helping the Spleen and Stomach do their job well too.

Relinquish your worries. Letting go of anything that makes you ruminate can help you relax your lips and turn a perpetual frown back into a smile.

Pay attention to your cravings for sweets. Have you been indulging too much? Your relationship with sugar will tell you if your Spleen is in trouble … and if your lips are too.

Chew your food well and refrain from eating before going to bed. When food is not well digested, imbalances in your Stomach and Spleen *Qi* are created that are reflected in the health of your smile.

The same is true when you work at your desk while eating lunch. The Spleen oversees your thought process as well as your digestion. Working and eating simultaneously splits the Spleen's focus, causing digestive problems and, in turn, distressed lips.

Massage the acupressure points shown in the following illustration to help stimulate your own collagen production. As a bonus, this massage will not only help reduce creases and lines in and around your lips, it will help rid you of other facial wrinkles too. Acupuncture treatments to these areas also promise noticeable results, so seek out the expertise of an acupuncturist near you.

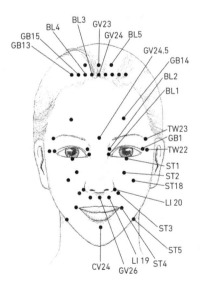

PATIENT-TESTED TRUTHS

I have a patient named Cindy who writes to me often between visits to let me know what is going on in her life. Her early notes mentioned her struggles with anxiety and its effect on her Stomach. What she didn't realize at the time is that anxiety and its associated Stomach issues tend to also impact the appearance of our lips, facial muscles, and flesh tone. Several weeks into her treatment, Cindy told me that her mother-in-law, whom she described as a "member in good standing of the plastic surgery club," had noticed how rejuvenated Cindy was looking and suspected she had "joined the club" as well. Of course, Cindy didn't undergo surgery. She was receiving acupuncture treatments to rid herself of the Stomach pain that always accompanied her anxiety. In the process, her lips and facial muscles were reaping the benefits too. Her mother-in-law's reaction naturally gave Cindy great encouragement. She came to me seeking acupuncture and mind-body techniques that could help her resolve her abdominal pains, but she loved the fact that the treatments were also improving the way she looked and felt emotionally. The treatments were a boon to her smile in more ways than she could have possibly known.

A WORD ABOUT THE TONGUE

While we are talking about the lips, we should probably talk a little bit about the tongue, as it is also a strong indicator of our health and beauty. In fact, the tongue is considered a distinguished diagnostic tool in Chinese medicine. It is the only internal organ that you can see from the outside. The tongue is called the *flame of the Heart* because the Heart supports it and also because it is considered an actual extension of the Heart.

Looking closely at its vessels, muscle, and nerve endings and considering its correlation to the Heart can tell practitioners volumes about how a patient is doing physically, emotionally, and intellectually.

For instance, the tongue's vessels indicate the health of one's blood. Look in the mirror and stick out your tongue. What color is it? Is that color evenly distributed?

Or are some parts darker or redder than others? Where are those dark spots located? Is there a film or coating on your tongue? What color and consistency is that coating? Is it thin, transparent, and a little white-ish? Or is the coating thick, greasy, and yellow in color? The answers to these questions all have very specific meanings.

Now raise your tongue. Do you see the veins beneath it? Are they dilated, congested, or barely visible at all? Whatever you observe here is happening to the veins throughout your body.

Your tongue will also indicate if your body is retaining excess fluids. Do you see ridges along the sides? When the tongue swells, it pushes against your teeth, leaving these notable indentations behind.

Does your tongue ever tremor or move around involuntarily? Your tongue is actually full of nerve endings, so its movement is connected to the brain through the Heart. Together, your tongue and voice articulate the words you think and feel. Their connection to the Heart and brain is why you experience slurred speech when you drink too much. Under the influence of alcohol your brain activity and speech functioning slows down considerably.

By contrast, when we say someone has a *clever tongue,* it means they are clear headed and witty—they are so in touch with what's in their heart they're able to give timely expression to those thoughts and feelings. In other words, command over your tongue usually means command over your cognitive and emotional functions.

Color, coating, swelling, motion, and shape are just some of the many indicators that practitioners of Chinese medicine are looking at when they examine your tongue. Each reveals something very specific about your Heart or the many other organs the tongue is connected to in some way.

Before we delve further into what some of these signs may mean, let's look at how the different parts of the tongue correspond with different organs:

- The back of the tongue is associated with the Kidneys and Bladder.
- The region between the back and center is associated with the Small and Large Intestines.

- The center is associated with the Spleen and Stomach.
- The region between the center and the tip is associated with the Lungs.
- The tip is associated with the Heart.
- The outer left ridge is associated with the Liver and the right ridge is associated with the Gallbladder.

All of this is made clearer in the illustration shown here.

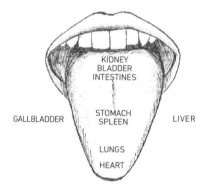

Note that the color of your tongue changes under a wide variety of conditions depending on any short- or long-term illnesses you may have, or even the time of year and whether Heat, Cold, Dampness, Dryness, or Wind *Qi* is prevalent during that season. It is difficult in just a few pages to interpret all the signs discussed earlier, but here is a brief explanation of what a few of the more common indicators suggest about your health:

Color

A normal tongue is pink. It is not too red or too pale.

A dark red tongue often indicates excessive Heat. You may feel warm all the time or you may sweat regardless of what the temperature is around you.

If the tip of the tongue is redder than the rest, this indicates excessive Heat in the Heart. Under these conditions you may have trouble with anxiety and insomnia.

A pale tongue often indicates deficient Blood *Qi*. You may feel lethargic throughout the day or generally bloated. You may even be light-headed, dizzy, or short of breath. It is wise to check your blood pressure if you experience these symptoms.

A purple tongue often indicates stagnated blood and *Qi* circulation. People who have this symptom can experience tightness and pain in the chest, shortness of breath, or pain in the upper abdomen and under the rib cage. Joint, ligament, and tendon pain will sometimes follow as well.

Coatings

Westerners tend to brush their tongues while brushing their teeth to keep their breath fresh, but they really shouldn't because they are blurring many vital clues about their overall health.

A thin white but transparent coating is normal. It should be clear enough to see the color of the tongue beneath the film.

A thick greasy coating concentrated in the middle of the tongue indicates excessive Dampness in the Spleen and Stomach. You may suffer from poor digestion and food stagnation. You may also experience weight gain and feel tired or listless as a result. When it is concentrated in the back third of the tongue, it indicates excessive Dampness in the Kidney and Bladder. You may also experience problems in the pelvic region, including urinary tract, yeast, and/or vaginal infections.

A thick yellow coating indicates that food that might have been stagnating in your digestive system has generated excessive *Yang* (Heating) energy. You may experience flatulence, body odor, or bad breath as a result.

A black or gray coating means there are internal toxicities and excessive Heat present. I have noticed that patients who have undergone chemotherapy for the treatment of cancer or those who had taken antibiotics for infection also tend to present a black or gray tongue coating.

A partial coating, or no coating at all, can mean that the Stomach's *Yin* (Cooling) energy is partially or totally deficient. Under these conditions people tend to experience excessive hunger, a thirst for cold drinks, and insomnia.

Movements

Of course, our tongue moves every time we speak, and most of us are fortunate to have total control over this movement. However, when the tongue becomes stiff and hard to move, it can reflect energetic dysfunctions involving multiple internal organs, particularly the Heart and the Liver. When the tongue tremors beyond one's control, as in the case of Parkinson's disease, it reflects excessive Wind energy due to deficient Liver *Yin* or Liver blood and requires acupuncture treatment and the use of herbs administered by a qualified practitioner to help correct this imbalance.

Other Common Indicators

A deepened crack down the center of the tongue indicates Deficient Essence.

A puffy tongue, with teeth marks lining the edges indicates water retention caused by Spleen, Kidney, and Lung *Qi* Deficiency.

Throughout this section, we've discussed several ways the tongue communicates with us on the subject of health. As you can see, the tongue's messages are not only numerous, they are replete with important information that can be used to help devise a treatment plan. **I don't expect you to be able to evaluate your own health by reading this section or by examining your tongue yourself. And I certainly don't expect you to arrive at a diagnosis of any kind.** I offer this perspective so you can use your tongue to speak up when and if you notice anything unusual happening with this organ because it means something unusual is likely to be occurring elsewhere in your body too. Examine your tongue periodically to see if it corroborates how you're feeling. If it appears different in any significant way than it typically does, then visit a Chinese medical practitioner near you.

I must say, it surprises me to this day that even though this organ provides an invaluable peek at our internal workings, Chinese medicine is the only form of medicine that reads peoples' tongues like this. It is yet another way in which this classical medicine excels over others.

Bear in mind that in Chinese medicine no single factor determines the course of action that will be recommended for you. The different signs just mentioned, as well as countless other factors, need to be taken into consideration before a course of treatment is decided upon. The body is such a highly nuanced system that two patients could come into our clinic complaining of the same symptoms and end up being treated in entirely different ways. The following cases are a direct example of this phenomenon.

PATIENT-TESTED TRUTHS

Kathy is a forty-five-year-old executive director of a nonprofit organization. She suffered from daily migraine headaches for more than twenty years. Her quality of life and her level of productivity at work suffered as a result. Multiple medications and supplements barely helped her get by. Her tongue looked pale and puffy and had tooth marks along the edges. The coating was thick and white. Her pulse was thin and wiry. Kathy apparently had Deficient Blood and *Qi* and excessively Cold energy that caused stagnation in her Liver and Gallbladder channels. A course of treatment with acupuncture and herbal remedies designed to replenish her *Qi* and blood, as well as remove the stagnation and warm up the meridians, significantly reduced her migraines.

Jacqueline, a fifty-year-old homemaker, also suffered from migraines over the course of the past fifteen years. However, a review of her tongue and an overall examination of her health told us a story different than Kathy's. Jacqueline's migraines were accompanied by depressed moods, bouts of insomnia, and abdominal pain. Her pulse was superficially strong and tense. Her tongue was red with purple spots and exhibited a fine tremor. It barely had any coating. The veins underneath her tongue were also congested. Although the two patients suffered from the same ailment, the cause of Jacqueline's migraines was different than Kathy's. Jacqueline's was prompted by a Liver *Yin* Deficiency with Liver *Yang* rising, in addition to Liver *Qi* and Blood Stagnation. A totally different strategy and treatment with acupuncture and Chinese herbal remedies were prescribed to help her.

The conditions that brought about each patient's headaches were markedly different; therefore each patient's treatment had to be customized uniquely for her. This is how complete a health assessment can be in Chinese medicine, and also how personal the solution tends to be.

As always, it's important for you to do all that you can to nurture your primary organs and to use all of the tools your own body provides (such as your tongue!) to help monitor your health and healing progress. When you do this, you will be doing all that you can to increase the odds of maintaining your long-term health and beauty. For more specific courses of action, work with your health-care practitioner.

Norma Muses on *Healthy Smiles and Smart Mouths*

For years—actually for most of my life—I wore red, red, red lipstick and red nail polish. I think I was born with red lipstick on. That was until Horst Rechelbacher, the Austrian-born hairstylist who educated so many of us in the 1990s about the toxic chemicals in many cosmetics, offered us such amazing alternatives through the companies he founded, including Aveda and, later, Intelligent Nutrients. Before reading his books and talking with him, I was unaware of the dangers of wearing lipstick, including ingesting it, as anybody who wears it does. To this day, there are many lipstick brands that contain cadmium, a carcinogen that appears in breast cancer biopsies and causes cancer cells to grow in controlled lab tests. And that's not the only toxic metal found in some popular brands. Lead, aluminum, chromium, and manganese among others have also been detected in recent studies. Lead is so dangerous it has been banned in paint and gasoline, yet it still exists in cosmetics most women wear all day long! There are studies identifying the pounds of lipstick women consume a year. This information is what made me switch to wearing plant-based stains only. There are so many beautiful new options to choose from now—options that still allow us to be girly girls without toxicity. It's really important that we learn to never put anything on our skin or lips that we wouldn't put in our mouth. And the same holds true for toothpaste, as many popular brands contain ingredients that cause hormone and environmental disruptions among other problems. For this reason I use a refreshing tooth soap that has no sugars, fluoride, or toxic chemicals. It's a simple blend of olive, coconut, and essential oils with distilled water. I freshen my mouth with a rinse that contains Himalayan salts, bicarb of soda, and whole-food calcium and magnesium along with essential oil. The brand I use has a citrusy flavor that has the added benefit of neutralizing acidity.

Of course, having learned from Dr. Yang how important a barometer of our health our lips and tongue are, I'm even happier to use these healthier products. Tooth soaps and natural rinses clean your teeth and balance the internal environment of your mouth without compromising the clues to your health that your tongue provides to you and your doctor. And because lip stains highlight, accentuate, and moisturize your lips rather than cake, cover up, or hide them, they permit the life of your smile to shine through for all to see. While our eyes do a lot of the talking in conversations with other people, as we discussed earlier, our lips obviously do too. A smile sends the first invitation to connect. It should be as genuine as possible.

HOW TO FIND A GOOD ACUPUNCTURIST AND CHINESE MEDICINE PRACTITIONER

Throughout this chapter there have been several times when I have recommended that you seek the expertise of a good Chinese medicine practitioner and acupuncturist, but you may wonder what exactly this task entails. The answer to this question is simple, especially now that you have read as much as you have about traditional Chinese medicine.

A good acupuncturist or Chinese medicine practitioner will recognize the anatomy and physiology of the human body just as modern medicine does, but he or she will also operate with the additional understanding of the human being's energetic network as mapped out for us by the ancients. As I described in great detail earlier, an acupuncturist works with Qi—the vital life force that keeps the body functioning physically and mentally—as well as with the different meridians that serve as the Qi's pathway to the major internal organs. They also recognize that any physical, chemical, or emotional stress will compromise the Qi and block the meridians, causing any number of abnormalities modern medicine calls *symptoms*.

Acupuncturists know all the specific points or tiny areas on the surface of the body that are connected with specific meridians and organ systems and can stimulate these points with the insertion and manipulation of fine needles. These needles open the blocked meridians and redirect the adequate flow of Qi to where it is intended.

Just like modern Western doctors, they can reduce the dysfunction and symptoms a patient is feeling. But they also *prevent* the symptoms from developing into serious illness and disease by the work they do even before the needles are inserted.

Their most important job is evaluating and diagnosing the meridians that are involved and determining the Qi that is imbalanced. The diagnosis and the Qi evaluation direct the selection of the points and the techniques of needling. This diagnostic process requires clinical skills, including reading the tongue and pulse, both of which are powerful diagnostic tools unique to Chinese medicine.

Although the symptoms and dysfunction may respond to the acupuncture treatment immediately after the first session, any chronic condition will require a course of daily treatment to achieve significant improvement. Bear in mind that American patients typically commit to only two or three sessions per week, but thirty sessions of treatment are typically needed to significantly improve most chronic conditions. **As you adopt this kind of care, realize that an investment of time up front can save you years and money in the long run!**

In addition to recognizing and addressing the causes of the *Qi* imbalance, a good acupuncturist will also provide tools for self-care and help patients make lifestyle modifications. As I have said before, you must always be an active partner in your own wellness plan.

Just as in choosing any professional to perform a service for you, referrals are important. The best types of referrals are ones from your friends and people you trust who have had a positive experience and outcome with a particular practitioner. If you don't know anyone who can refer you to a practitioner, you can find listings online, including one on the Tao Institute of Mind and Body Medicine website. Be sure to meet and interview any practitioner you are considering before undergoing treatment. Let your intuition and the answers to your questions be your guide. Ask them how they diagnose their patients and what their treatment plan entails. You may also want to ask what their experience has been in treating conditions like yours. Don't be afraid to ask for clarification when you don't understand something. **Doctors must be teachers too, especially as your own involvement is an important factor in the long-term success of the treatment.**

The bottom line is that you want to see if they care about their work and their patients and if they are confident about what they know. A good acupuncturist will use acupuncture as a tool to attend to the complete health of the body, rather than as a needle to simply simulate the skin, muscles, or nerves in service to the anatomy alone. They are no different from any other health-care professional in that they must have a caring heart, sound knowledge, evident clinical skills, and the ability to communicate effectively. And they especially need to be able to develop a therapeutic alliance with their patients.

In addition, a good acupuncturist must be able to appreciate the energetic system of the human being as ancient Chinese medicine describes. Because there are no external tools that make it possible to see this system, the practitioner has to be able to visualize it armed with a combination of knowledge, experience, and what I like to call *quantum glasses*—spectacles that have not yet been invented but which enable us to see objects on a quantum level. Understanding the energetic nature of a human being is critical for the treatment process. The human body is an open system that constantly exchanges its energy with that of the natural environment and people around it. This person should advise patients to be mindful of their surrounding climate changes, behaviors, and interpersonal relationships. Norma and I are teaching you some of these awareness skills throughout this book, but they will only be honed with practice.

Since energy circulates in the meridian systems in an orderly and timely fashion, the acupuncturist should encourage patients to live a life congruent with the energetic flow of nature. This includes providing clear instruction on a good time to rise, rest, exercise, eat, and cleanse.

An acupuncturist's own energy is also important when interacting and intervening with the energy of the patient. A good acupuncturist cultivates his or her energy to a healthy level and remains very focused during the treatment.

Finding such a partner, and reading this book to make you an informed patient, will go a long way toward helping to bring you the kind of inner and outer health you clearly desire.

Other Common Treatment Modalities in Chinese Medicine

It might also help for you to become familiar with some of the more common treatment modalities in Chinese medicine before you meet and interview your practitioner. Next you will find descriptions of the practices you may encounter in addition to acupressure and acupuncture.

Cupping: This treatment stimulates the flow of blood and energy and helps to eliminate toxins, cellular waste, and excess fluid from the region being worked on. It involves burning a swab of cotton inside a glass cup to warm it. When the cup is placed upside-down over a specific area of the patient's body, it creates a vacuum. As the cup is lifted, the resulting suction draws the skin upward, gently massaging it and helping to release any impurities.

Moxibustion: Much like cupping, this practice invigorates the circulation of both blood and *Qi*. It involves burning a cone-shaped piece of moxa on a specific acupuncture point. Moxa is made from the Asian mugwort herb, which is known to heal people with Cold or stagnant *Qi*. The patient will experience a pleasant warm sensation as the herb's heat penetrates the skin. The cone is typically extinguished before it can burn the patient. Alternatively, the practitioner might light one end of a moxa stick, which resembles a cigar, and hold it close to the area being treated for several minutes in lieu of actually letting the moxa rest on the skin. Depending upon the condition being treated, there are also instances when an acupuncture needle wrapped in moxa is lit and inserted into an acupuncture point, delivering Heat to the point that way.

Customized herbal remedies: These include a wide range of herbal treatments, the ingredients of which are specially selected and mixed by a practitioner who takes into account all of the patient's unique energy needs. Various herbs are strategically combined to enhance their efficacy, minimize any potential side effects, and eliminate toxicity. They are often prepared as decoctions, bullet-like pills, powders, or capsules. They are typically taken on an empty stomach, with warm or hot water, and two times daily. The formula should be reviewed and modified every ten or twenty days to keep apprised of the body's changing energetic status.

Tui na: *Tui na* is yet another manual therapy based on the principles and understanding of human *structural and energetic anatomy, physiology, and functionality* within Chinese medicine. Its numerous techniques involve applying pressure on select acupuncture points, massaging the body along the involved meridians, pulling and pushing the muscles and extremities of the body, as well as stretching and rotating joints.

Gua sha: *Gua sha* is a convenient tool for home and self-care. It involves repeated pressured strokes and scrapes over lubricated skin with a smooth edge, such as a soup spoon, honed animal bones, water buffalo horn, or jade. Again it is based on the evaluation of involved meridians and organs predicated on Chinese medicine theories, and it works on the acupuncture points and meridians. It helps eliminate toxins and remove stagnation of blood and *Qi*. Dark and sand-like bruises appear as result of the treatment, and as evidence of the underlying problems. I recall successfully providing this treatment on my father under his instruction starting when I was fifteen years old and once a year thereafter as a part of his overall health management.

Congratulations, you are now ready to seek out, interview, and secure a qualified Chinese medicine practitioner and partner in creating your own personal wellness plan.

11

A Regimen for All Seasons

CARING FOR YOURSELF YEAR-ROUND

Because of my work I think about the ways the seasons relate to our bodies all the time. A true lifestyle collection must adapt to many changing factors, not the least of which are climate and weather conditions, because women really live in their clothes. Creating timeless style—not just fashion, but *real* fashion—is contingent on this. It's more than aiming to keep people warm in the winter and cool in the summer, and offering the maximum number of options in the spring and fall when conditions are less extreme but also less consistent. It's about navigating the many transitions that occur within a given day—that's how intimately we all relate to the seasons. **Dr. Yang, I know that the seasons are an extremely important factor in Chinese medicine too, so what wisdom can you share to help us all weather them better in terms of health and beauty?**

There is no denying that the seasons have a profound effect on us. We all know that strong winds and bright sunshine can be damaging to the eyes; Dry Heat can be the kiss of death for skin and lips; and humidity can wreak havoc with our hair. But the seasons also have a far greater impact on us. As you've delved deeper and deeper into this book, I'm sure you've begun to notice that the body experiences a kind of *sensory inundation* every day. All that we look at, hear, taste, smell, and feel influences our overall health, our outer appearance, as well as how we think and function in life.

Visualized at the energetic level, the human body is in constant interaction with energy from the environment. Our bodies are in dialogue and exchange with Cold, Heat, Dampness, Dryness, and/or Wind all of the time. **Some of these energies are more prevalent and excessive during one season than another so what we do to balance our interactions with them really varies by time of year.**

When you look at the changing conditions from season to season and the ways we try to help our bodies adjust to them, you cannot help but see the theory of *Yin* and *Yang* at work. Being our most vital and beautiful selves year-round is all about maintaining balance between the external and internal environments. Let's examine the seasons together, focusing on how to protect ourselves when these outside forces impact our bodies, as well as how to proactively use what is available to us in our environment to nurture our bodies and maintain or restore our youthful good looks.

As you will recall from chapter 2, Chinese medicine teaches us that each season is associated with a different *Qi:*

- The **spring** is most strongly associated with **Wind**.
- The **summer** is most strongly associated with **Heat**.
- The **late summer** is most strongly associated with **Dampness**.
- The **fall** is most strongly associated with **Dryness**.
- The **winter** is most strongly associated with **Cold**.

Chinese medicine also teaches us that specific organs are more vulnerable at different times of year and that exposure to the *Qi* most prevalent at that time can pose considerable challenges for those organs. For instance:

In the **spring** the **Liver and Gallbladder** are most vulnerable; therefore
everything along their meridian is too, including our nails, tendons,

ligaments, eyes, vision, and tear flow. So too are our digestion, menstruation, judgment, decision-making abilities, and level of emotional sensitivity.

During this fertile season, it's the Wind's job to carry seeds and spores to where they will ultimately grow as vegetation. But the Wind also happens to carry Cold, Heat, Dampness, Dryness, bacteria, viruses, and other airborne pathogens with it. Because it can combine with these other pathogens in many different ways, it can cause a wide range of imbalances, conditions, and diseases once it enters the human body. It can be responsible for everything from colds, flus, sinusitis, earaches, a stiff neck, sore throat, coughing, itchy and sore eyes, skin rashes, dizziness, blurred vision, headaches, and toothaches. It can also cause spasms and bone and muscle pain, and it can exacerbate chronic illnesses such as epilepsy, Parkinson's disease, and stroke among other conditions.

In the **summer** the **Heart and Small Intestine** are most vulnerable; therefore everything along their meridian is too, including our complexion, pulse, veins, arteries, tongue, and speech. So too is our ability to regulate sweat, circulate blood, take initiative, communicate effectively, and exercise good conscience, spirituality, and overall creativity.

During this season of increased and often unrelenting Heat, the body can experience everything from fever, throat irritation, cough with phlegm, headaches, skin rashes, conjunctivitis, and sinus infections to excessive thirst, constipation, reduced urine output, increased sweating, heat stroke, irregular heartbeat, anxiety, and insomnia among many other symptoms, diseases, and conditions depending upon where the Heat ends up residing and with which other pathogens it joins forces.

In the **late summer** the **Spleen and Stomach** are most vulnerable; therefore everything along their meridian is too, including our lips, flesh, muscles, mouth, and sense of taste. So too is our ability to maintain our body's defenses, to regulate our saliva, absorption, digestion, and metabolism, and to think, reason, and maintain a strong sense of clarity.

During this season, frequently noted for its humidity and Dampness, the body's hair and skin can become oily, leading to acne and other skin eruptions. The body can also experience mucus buildup in the nasal passages and elsewhere. One tends to feel heavy in the limbs, foggy in the brain, and swollen in the joints. Diarrhea, poor appetite, indigestion, water retention, and weight gain are also more likely to occur during this season. Women may experience more vaginal discharge with or without odor as well. Dampness can foster Heat if it is not treated soon enough. Damp Heat often causes swelling, redness, and pain in the affected part of the body, similar to what we see in all kinds of conditions featuring inflammation and infection, such as inflammatory bowel diseases, rheumatoid arthritis, acute hepatitis, and candida, among others.

In the **fall** the **Lungs and Large Intestine** are most vulnerable; therefore everything along their meridian is too, including our body hair and skin, nose and sense of smell. So too is our ability to regulate our breathing, how much mucus we generate, how much water we retain, and what levels of discipline, restraint, and intuition we can sustain.

During this season when arid conditions prevail, we will often experience dry hair, eyes, mouth, throat, and nasal passages, chapped skin and lips, fever, headache, excessive thirst, nosebleeds, dry cough, dry stools, and/or reduced urine output.

In the **winter** the **Kidneys and Urinary Bladder** are most vulnerable; therefore everything along their meridian is too, including the health of our hair, bones, and hearing. So too is our ability to regulate our urine output, our physical growth and development, our reproductive and sexual functions as well as the degree of willpower, motivation, and coordination we exhibit, not to mention our level of spontaneity.

During this season of consistently cold temperatures, the body can struggle to stay warm. The blood may stagnate, causing pain in the joints and lower back. You may even experience a stiff neck caused by drafts. The Cold can also cause fever with chills, headaches, sneezing and a runny nose, loose stools, poor digestion, abdominal pain, bloating, fatigue, a slowed pulse, discolored lips, fingers, and toes, as well as black circles under your eyes. The Cold is also associated with joint pain, skeletal muscular pain, sciatic and other nerve pain, hernias, muscle strain and pulls, testicular pain, and sperm production challenges in men, as well as menstrual cramps in women.

WAYS TO PROTECT YOUR *QI* BY SEASON

Certainly, to help you achieve balance between the outer and internal energies that exist in any given season, you should minimize your exposure to the prevalent pathogen in that season, and you should also maximize your care and attention to the most vulnerable organs at that time. Bear in mind that if you live in a climate where Wind, Heat, Dampness, Dryness, or Cold is prevalent for more than one-fifth of the year—or, in some cases, year-round—you should feel free to apply the following tips in those extended seasons as necessary.

Also, as you read through the suggestions offered here, think about the results of the evaluation you completed at the outset of this book, which was designed to help you determine your general energetic constitution. If you are prone to internal Dampness, Heat, Cold, Dryness, or stagnation as indicated by this evaluation, consult a practitioner about how you might make extra efforts to achieve energetic balance during the seasons that will likely challenge you most. (If you like, now is a good time to turn to the Appendix and score your results for a more accurate picture of your personal energetic constitution!)

In the **spring** bear in mind all the steps described in this book so far to nurture your Liver and Gallbladder, including but not limited to releasing any anger you may be feeling or grudges you may be harboring from recent or past events; wearing a wooden accessory or the color cyan to allow their energies to fortify you; and by protecting your eyes, nails, tendons, and ligaments against harsh winds. Caring for your Liver and Gallbladder may also mean:

Keeping all the joints of your legs and arms well covered.

Wearing sunglasses or dabbing some rose or jasmine oil on your pulse points as a way of barring the Wind's entry into your body.

Staying out of the path of drafts from open windows, vents, fans, and air conditioners (the latter of which many of us are tempted to use on the first unseasonably warm day before they have even been properly cleaned).

Pursuing acupuncture as well as cupping and customized herbal remedies.

Massaging the following acupuncture points to help sedate and dispel Wind from the body: LIV3, GB20, LU9, LI 11, LI 4, KID1, SP6.

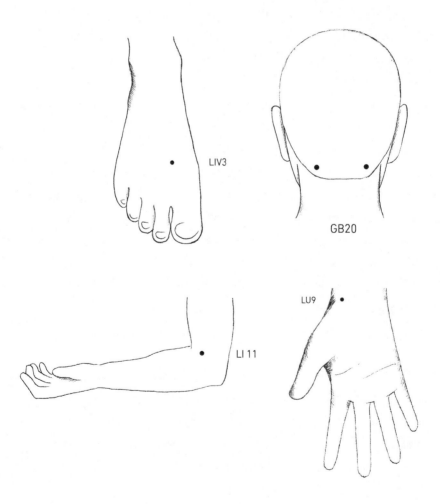

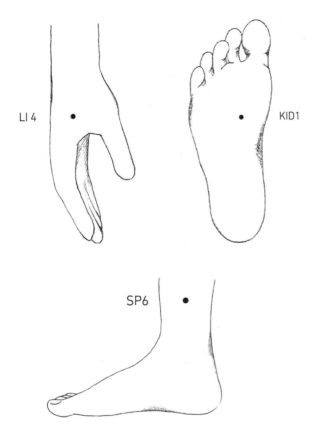

Other ways to balance the *Yin* and *Yang* energies within your body during the springtime include paying attention to what you eat, making a special effort to add sour-tasting foods to your diet such as some of the foods listed on the Seasonal Shopping List provided on page 158. A word to the wise: These are general guidelines, so be sure to check with your practitioner before making any major dietary changes and *don't* overindulge. Chinese medicine is based on the concept of balance. If your practitioner agrees, pick and choose a few items from this food list. Swap in different ones every day to maintain variety. Also note that if you eat too many sour-tasting foods to support your Liver you can potentially overwhelm your Spleen, causing water retention and stiff ligaments.

147

Remember our discussion of the Theory of Five Elements in chapter 4 in which I explained how Wood overcomes Earth. The Liver is a Wood organ and can easily overcome the Spleen, an Earth organ, if you eat far too many sour foods. So eat just enough to nurture your liver without going overboard. Also avoid pungent foods as they tend to counteract the benefits of sour foods.

In the **summer** bear in mind the steps described up to this point to nurture your Heart and Small Intestine, including embracing the joy in your life; speaking to others honestly and *from the heart;* wearing red and its lighter shades such as pink and cerise to help naturally regulate the Heat in your body; minding what you say (definitely not getting *too hot-tempered*); monitoring your pulse; noting how flushed your complexion may be getting; and watching how much you're perspiring, all as a way to help guard against the Heat. Caring for your Heart and Small Intestine may also mean:

Keeping your environment well ventilated to help regulate your sweat.

Avoiding excessive use of air-conditioning.

Receiving acupuncture treatments focused on nurturing and balancing Qi in the Heart and Small Intestine.

Applying acupressure on the following acupuncture points: HT8, HT3, SI 2, SI 8, KID2, KID10, BL63, LIV2.

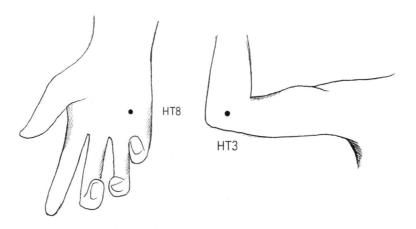

HT8

HT3

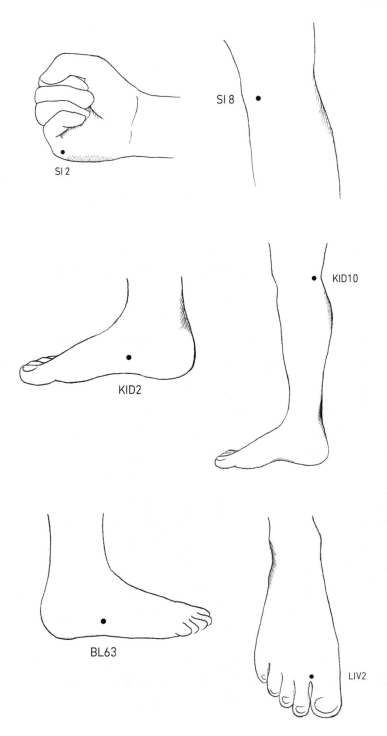

SI 8

SI 2

KID10

KID2

BL63

LIV2

Quenching your thirst with only select beverages. Most people think ice-cold drinks cool them down in the heat of the summer, but the truth is, *sweating* is what cools us. The purpose of drinking when we're hot is to help replenish the fluids we lose while perspiring. In fact, chilled beverages congeal your *Qi* and keep it from flowing as readily as it should. While it sounds counterintuitive, you really should avoid cold fluids altogether, including many of your summertime favorites from frosted mugs of beer, Margaritas and other frozen cocktails, iced lattes, and cold sodas to thick smoothies and milkshakes. Stick with room-temperature water to satisfy your thirst. It really is the most natural solution. Warm or room-temperature green tea—as opposed to iced tea—imparts cooling energy too, and has the added bonus of delivering rich antioxidants to your system.

Other ways to balance the *Yin* and *Yang* energies within your body during the summer include paying attention to what you eat, making a special effort to add bitter-tasting foods to your diet, and enjoying more cooling foods such as duck, crabmeat, fish, tofu, celery, lotus roots, tomatoes, wax gourd, bitter melon, watermelon, lychee, plums, strawberries, apples, and apricots. These foods generally provide increased fluids to your body and help replenish what is lost through sweat. Many of these foods appear on the Seasonal Shopping List provided on page 158. The same advice I offered earlier applies here as well—see your practitioner before making any major dietary changes and don't overindulge in the foods on this list. Pick and choose a few items. Eating too many bitter-tasting foods to support your Heart will overwhelm your Lungs and cause damage to your skin and body hair. In our discussion of the Theory of Five Elements in chapter 4, we talked about how Fire overcomes Metal. The Heart, as a Fire organ, can overcome the Lungs, a Metal organ, if you eat bitter foods in excess, so eat just enough to nurture your Heart, not to harm your Lungs. Also avoid salty foods as they tend to neutralize the benefits of bitter foods.

In the **late summer** bear in mind the steps described up to this point to nurture your

Spleen and Stomach, including but not limited to freeing yourself of worries and doubts, and stretching your muscles to help keep them injury free as you engage in outdoor fun. Caring for your Spleen and Stomach may also mean:

Taking precautions to keep your skin dry and free of ringworm or athlete's foot after showering, swimming, jogging, or participating in any other sport.

Cleaning the surfaces of your home and office with tea tree oil to naturally and safely remove mold and mildew.

Wearing the color yellow so its warm energies can help evaporate the Dampness around you.

Wearing loose-fitting clothing to keep the body well ventilated and to prevent Dampness from getting trapped close to the pores of your skin. Again, natural fabrics such as hemp, linen, and cotton are ideal.

Many of the people who see me during this time of year are also helped by such treatments as cupping and moxibustion, which were described in chapter 10. Herbal wraps, which involve the application of poultices to swollen joints to help draw out any fluids that may be causing edema, also work wonders, as does acupuncture.

In the absence of these treatments, you might also opt to place a heating pad on your joints or to gently massage the following acupressure points to help expel Dampness: SP9, SP3, ST40, LI 2, LU9, HT7, SI 2, GV20.

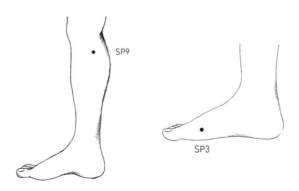

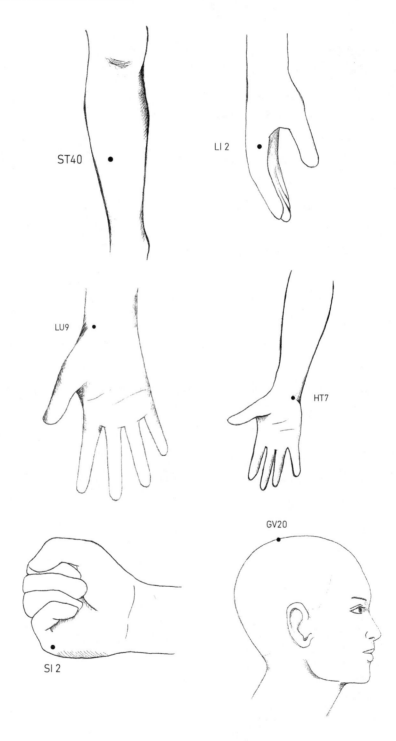

Other ways to balance the *Yin* and *Yang* energies within your body in the late summer include making a special effort to add sweet-tasting foods to your diet. A few of these are listed on the Seasonal Shopping List on page 158. Once again, don't get overzealous. Check in with your practitioner first for a full evaluation. With their approval, pick and choose only a few items from this food list. Eating too many sweet-tasting foods to support your Spleen will increase Dampness in your muscles; block the flow of Qi to your Stomach, thereby slowing the digestive process; and will also overwhelm your Kidneys, causing your hair to fall out and your bones to ache. You will recall that in our discussion of the Theory of Five Elements in chapter 4, Earth dams Water. The Spleen, as an Earth organ, can overcome the Kidneys, a Water organ, if you eat sweet foods in excess. So eat just enough to nurture your Spleen without injuring your Lungs. Also avoid sour-tasting foods, as they tend to counteract the benefits of sweet foods. Your practitioner may also suggest:

Adding the zest from the peel of lemons, limes, or oranges when grilling beef to help reduce its Dampness quotient.

Refraining from eating greasy foods despite the time-honored American tradition of enjoying fried chicken at this time of year. Greasy foods are not easily metabolized in the late summer and also contribute to increased internal Dampness.

Reducing the amount of dairy in your diet for the same reasons. Yes, that means ice cream!

Introducing more cooked foods to help the digestive system work best even though fresh salads seem most tempting during these months. Cooked vegetables also provide a better supply of methyl groups for an important biochemical process called methylation. Essentially, methylation allows us to make, maintain, and repair our own DNA. It works by shutting down the activity of genes that cause hereditary disease and green-lighting the activity of genes that promote our health.

Eating smaller meals for the same reason.

Starting a new summer tradition in the name of health and beauty by adding warm soups to your diet to reduce Dampness. Warm broth-based soups are a staple in the Chinese diet and should become part of your regular meal plan too.

In the **fall** bear in mind the steps described up to this point to nurture your Lungs and Large Intestine, including but not limited to moving on from feelings of loss, grief, or sadness as much as possible. Unfortunately, the fall is often the time when people move away from family and friends or from a city they love, changing schools or jobs, or making other major life decisions that can leave them longing for the way things used to be. If you have to make such changes, be sure you are well prepared mentally and emotionally, and that you process your feelings of loss and grief, taking measures to reduce them by staying in close contact with those you care about; wearing the color white and/or jewelry made from precious metals such as silver or gold for their cleansing and healing properties; keeping your nose and sinus passages naturally free and clear by humidifying your home or bedroom; and keeping your skin and body hair healthy by avoiding long, hot, drying showers and by eating foods rich in natural oils.

Other ways to balance the *Yin* and *Yang* energies within your body during the **fall** include paying attention to what you eat, making a special effort to add pungent-tasting foods to your diet. A few of these are listed on the Seasonal Shopping List provided on page 158. Once again, I encourage you to consult your practitioner first. Upon his or her recommendations, use pungent foods to help nurture your Lungs, but I caution you not to eat too many of them. Pick and choose a few items. Eating an excessive amount of pungent tasting foods to support your Lungs can damage your Liver, and your nails, tendons, and ligaments by extension. Again, according to the Theory of the Five Elements,

Metal overcomes Wood. The Lungs, as a Metal organ, can overcome the Liver, a Wood organ, if you eat pungent foods in excess, so eat just enough pungent foods to nurture your Lungs, and not enough to harm your Liver. Also avoid bitter foods as they tend to counteract the benefits of pungent foods. Your practitioner may also recommend:

Drinking room-temperature water as often as you can to hydrate your body.

Avoiding coffee and soda, as they tend to do the opposite.

Eating avocado, salmon, flax, and kelp, which will naturally help to keep your body well oiled and functioning properly.

Applying acupressure on the following acupuncture points: LU9, LI 11, KID7, SP6, ST36.

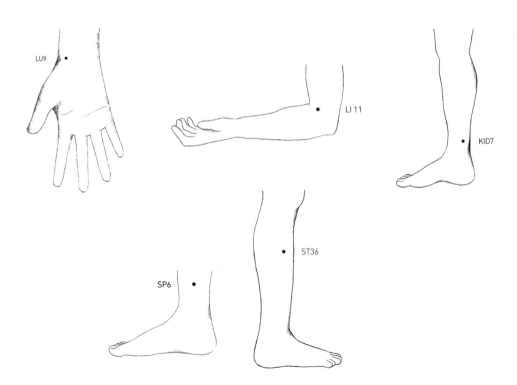

In the **winter** bear in mind the steps described up to this point to nurture your Kidneys and Urinary Bladder, including but not limited to letting go of fears, anxieties, and limiting thoughts; keeping your bones well covered and your joints safe from the Wind and Cold when outdoors; doing the same for your ears and massaging them too as a means of sending invigorating energies to the organs most taxed by the frigid weather; and finally, brushing your hair well each day to increase blood circulation just beneath the scalp.

Other ways to balance the *Yin* and *Yang* energies within your body during the **winter** include paying attention to what you eat, making a special effort to add salty-tasting foods to your diet. A few of these are listed on the Seasonal Shopping List provided on page 158. As always, get a full evaluation from your practitioner before making any dietary changes. Eating salty foods can potentially help nurture your Kidneys, but it is important to consider all other factors beforehand. Eating an excessive amount of salty foods to support your Kidneys can damage your Heart, causing Blood Stasis and blood-vessel blockage. As the Theory of Five Elements explains, Water overcomes Fire. The Kidneys, as a Water organ, can overcome the Heart, a Fire organ, under those circumstances, so eat just enough to nurture your Kidneys and not enough to extinguish your Heart Fire. Also avoid sweet foods as they tend to counteract the benefits of salty foods. Finally, your practitioner may also recommend:

Eating the kinds of food that help you store energy. These are foods typically higher in essential fatty acids and protein content.

Taking ginseng, rhemannia root, or astragalus remedies to increase your Kidney, Lung, and Liver energy and to help offset the kinds of food cravings we tend to have as we try to refuel and warm our bodies during one of the toughest seasons of the year to endure.

Applying acupressure on the following acupuncture points: KID3, KID6, LI 4, LI 11, HT3, HT7, SI 3, GV20.

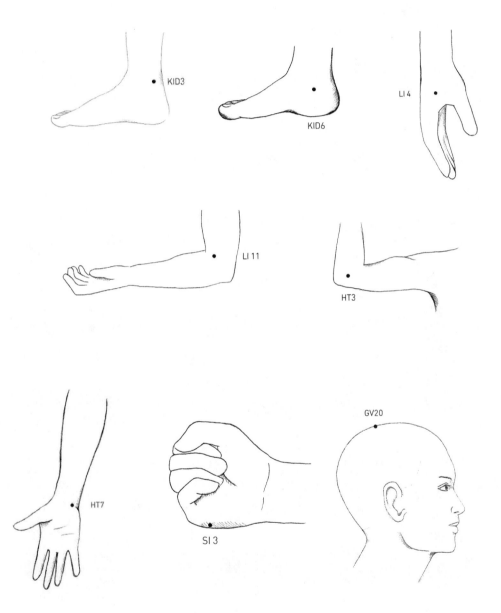

KID3

KID6

LI 4

LI 11

HT3

HT7

SI 3

GV20

YOUR SEASONAL SHOPPING LIST

If it's true that you are what you eat, consuming particular foods when they are most needed by your body means that you are well on your way to being your healthiest self year-round. The following is a list of groceries by season that, with proper guidance, can help you meet this goal.

FOODS FOR THE SPRING MONTHS WHEN WIND IS PREVALENT

VEGETABLES:

- Cabbage
- Celery
- Collards
- Green beans
- Iceberg lettuce
- Kale
- Onions
- Spinach

FRUITS:

- Dark plums*
- Green grapes
- Green olives
- Kiwi
- Lemon

OTHER:

- Azuki beans*
- Chicken*
- Chives*
- Seaweed

Practitioners often recommend these specific foods when patients have a Liver Qi Deficiency.

FOODS FOR THE SUMMER MONTHS WHEN HEAT IS PREVALENT

VEGETABLES:

- Artichokes
- Asparagus
- Beets
- Belgian endive
- Cucumbers
- Eggplant
- Lettuce
- Okra
- Radishes
- Red peppers
- Shelling beans
- Sweet peppers
- Tomatoes

FRUITS:

- Apricots*
- Blackberries
- Blueberries
- Cherries
- Figs
- Grapefruit

- Melons
- Nectarines
- Peaches

- Plums
- Pluots
- Raspberries

- Red-skinned apples
- Rhubarb
- Strawberries

OTHER:
- *Allium chinense* (Chinese onion)*

- Barley*
- Lamb*

- Wheat*

Practitioners often recommend these specific foods when patients have a Heart Qi Deficiency.

FOODS FOR THE LATE SUMMER MONTHS WHEN DAMPNESS IS PREVALENT

VEGETABLES:
- Bok choy
- Brussels sprouts
- Carrots
- Celeriac
- Corn

- Garlic
- Leeks
- Onions
- Parsnips
- Pumpkin

- Sweet potatoes
- Summer squash
- Turnips
- Yams
- Zucchini

FRUITS:
- Apples
- Bananas
- Figs
- Hawthorns

- Lemons
- Lychee
- Oranges
- Papaya

- Peaches
- Pomegranates

OTHER:
- Anchovies
- Beef
- Chestnuts
- Chickpeas

- Chinese dates*
- Cinnamon
- Coconuts
- Ginger

- Japanese rice*
- Malva crispa*
- Spelt
- Sugar cane

Practitioners often recommend these specific foods when patients have a Spleen Qi Deficiency.

FOODS FOR THE FALL MONTHS WHEN DRYNESS IS PREVALENT

VEGETABLES:
- Belgian endive
- Broccoli
- Brussels sprouts
- Cabbage
- Cauliflower
- Celeriac
- Lotus roots
- Lotus seeds
- Onions
- Pumpkins
- Spinach
- Squash
- Sweet potatoes
- Turnips
- Yams
- Zucchini

FRUITS:
- Apples
- Figs
- Grapes
- Peaches*

OTHER:
- Grains*
- Green onions*
- Venison (deer meat)*

Practitioners often recommend these specific foods when patients have a Lung Qi Deficiency.

FOODS FOR THE WINTER MONTHS WHEN COLD IS PREVALENT

VEGETABLES:
- *Allium chinense* (Chinese onion)
- Black mushrooms
- Cabbage
- Celery
- Chives
- Garlic
- Onions
- Potatoes
- Sweet potatoes
- Squash
- Turnips

FRUITS:
- Apples
- Asian pears
- Carambolas
- Kumquats
- Longans
- Quinces
- Rambutans
- Persimmons

OTHER:

- Bean sprouts*
- Black sesame seeds
- Chestnuts*
- Pork*
- Soybeans*

Practitioners often recommend these specific foods when patients have a Kidney Qi Deficiency.

As always, remember that while these foods are listed by the season in which they are needed most, you should feel free to eat foods that nurture a specific organ whenever that organ requires additional care no matter what time of year it is!

STILL MORE HEALTHY STEPS YOU CAN TAKE EACH SEASON!

The amount and type of **exercise** you engage in; the frequency with which you have **sex;** and the time and quality of your **sleep** can also greatly influence how you balance your *Qi* and how you protect and enhance your health and beauty throughout the year. Let's look at each of these factors individually.

About Exercise by Season

It is universally understood that exercise is an important part of our existence. We are, after all, animals. We were designed to move around. That's how life is supposed to be. If we don't keep in motion, everything in us will stagnate and rot. We were intended to exercise for more than just the development of muscle and the burning of fat. We were meant to exercise to insure that our *Qi* remains active. Exercise is not only vital for our muscles, bones, and joints; it is vital for the maintenance of our energy supply and our essence over time. Exercise helps us keep the meridians free and clear of blockages. When energy is not getting to its destination on time or in peak condition, we experience dysfunction—or worse—illness. When it is traveling according to schedule and delivering the highest-quality *Qi*, we are our best and brightest selves, inside and out.

The challenge is that many Westerners engage in exercise that is vigorous and highly repetitive. It often focuses on one *problem* area, but there is no balance or harmony in stressing a single part of our body repeatedly to its detriment and the detriment of other body parts. Our bodies are designed for a *variety* of movements that involve our whole being—our mind and spirit too. If you maintain an exercise regimen that is repetitive and mindless for a very long period of time, it is likely that you will require surgery in your life to replace a hip or knee or whatever other body part you wore down with such repetition. Whatever exercise you choose, try to develop an awareness of how energy moves in and around you. Pursuits such as meditation, tai chi, qigong, yoga, and even dance can help you do that. So too can a walk for thirty minutes a day. It doesn't need to be a particularly brisk walk. You simply have to practice a fluid activity that will keep your overall *Qi* circulating without straining individual muscles, tendons, or ligaments. With time you will become very attuned to both inner and outer energies, and you can adjust your routine to fit your body's needs.

To get you started, let me share with you some exercises that work in harmony with the external energies that exist in each given season.

Spring: Most people's energy is naturally robust during this season of rebirth and revitalization, so it is a good time to begin a regular exercise routine if you don't already have one. As mentioned earlier, walking for a half hour after meals, or between sedentary activities, or even on your way to or from work, is an ideal exercise that can easily fit into your schedule. Tai chi, qigong, yoga, dance, or meditation, as mentioned, are also wonderful choices. If you choose something different from these suggestions, note that it should *not* be something that makes you perspire too much, as this opens the pores to the Wind and the pathogens it carries.

Summer: The energy you typically feel during the spring tends to wane as the temperatures rise in the summer. Take precautions to protect the Heart from burning too intensely throughout this season. If you don't walk or partake in tai chi, yoga, qigong, meditation, or dance as suggested earlier, water sports offer a cooling balance to summer Heat. When swimming, be sure to vary your strokes so you are working different parts of your body. Despite the temptations to play other typical summer sports, resist any that might cause you to perspire excessively, as again, heavy exertion that brings about sweating causes the body to expend valuable *Qi* and Heart *Yang*.

Late summer: Since Dampness can make your whole chest feel heavy, participating in any activity that encourages deep breathing can help clear the body—particularly the Lungs—of excess moisture. This is the one time of year when perspiring in moderation is okay, as it will help rid your body of unwanted fluids. However, you must remember that Dampness is more often accompanied by Heat during these months, so you should still be sure not to overexert yourself. Enjoying the sauna at your gym may be the way to go this season: it can help remove toxins and excess fluids from your body without taxing your Heart *Yang* the way heavy exercise does. Playing a round of beach volleyball is another possibility. The dry, hot sand beneath your feet can help draw excess moisture out of your body too.

Fall: The fall is associated with the Lungs, so once again, any exercises that encourage deep breathing and motion are highly recommended. You know my often-recommended favorite activities already—tai chi, qigong, and yoga among others—though I might add martial arts to the list. These forms of exercise require an understanding of *Yin* and *Yang* especially as they relate to using motion and energy inside and outside of our bodies effectively.

Winter: This is the season to conserve energy, to store it up for the spring when a burst of new activity will require it most. Winter is usually the time when you bring your exercise routine indoors, but as you renew your gym membership, be sure to look for places that offer more than just the same kinds of repetitive exercises I addressed earlier. Engage in some light resistance training as this is important for toning and keeping muscles healthy, but also be sure to pursue exercises that circulate *Qi* throughout your entire body. Spinning or elliptical workouts can accomplish this goal as long as you design your routine to invigorate your upper body too. Yoga, tai chi, qigong, dance, and/or meditation continue to be preferred exercises. And on days when the rapidly dropping temperatures make it prohibitive to take long walks in nature, remember that there are other options to explore as well. One of my patients told me that she has seen people walking laps at our local shopping mall early in the morning before the stores open and the foot traffic builds. Now that kind of ingenuity is an example of *exercising* your mind too! I also try to take stairs more frequently during this season.

About Sex by Season

We talked in earlier chapters about how Kidney *Qi* and *Jing* (essence) is responsible for many things, among them our sexual functioning, including the capacity to procreate. So you already know that our Kidneys help us preserve life, and that they also help us give life, provided we conserve and use that *Qi* effectively.

When Chinese medicine addresses our sexuality more specifically in the context of the seasons, it actually teaches us all about the best times and conditions under which to expend that essence and energy.

That's right—there are seasons that are more conducive for lovemaking than others. The prevailing conditions in these seasons enable us to better balance *Yin* and *Yang* so they don't cost us as much *Qi* or essence as other seasons might.

Here's how it works:

The **spring** is when our sexual energies tend to be at their highest. This season represents a period of fertility in the natural cycle of life. It follows the winter, a season of rest. If you have nurtured your Kidneys during the wintertime as recommended, then the spring is an ideal time to engage in more regular sexual activity. As with every season, however, you should be careful to refrain on days when weather conditions are extreme (i.e., when there is heavy rain or fog.) If the spring comes in like a lion, then you know which days I am talking about. They usually fall in the first half of the season. Such weather conditions can affect the quantity of Kidney Qi that is released during intercourse. This is a wonderful time of year to enjoy sex as long as you are careful to avoid the days that will exhaust your Kidney essence, as lost essence causes some of the most deep-rooted *and* visible signs of aging.

The **summer** is the time of the year when everything is lush. Ripe fruits and vegetables are bursting with juice and even people glisten with sweat. These are all indications of how easy it is to release too many fluids from our bodies during these months. The Heat of this season suggests that you enjoy sexual activity, but in moderation, especially on the hottest of days. Valuable Qi is already escaping your body as you perspire throughout the day so you will want to be careful not to lose much more of it through excessive sexual activity.

The **late summer** poses less of a threat, but again I would caution you to pay attention to extreme weather conditions. Making love during a late summer lightning or thunderstorm can sap you of your Kidney essence even if the rest of the season is kinder to you.

The **fall** is the season when our bodies are notably the driest. It is a season that warrants retaining as much of your Qi as you can, so again, enjoy sex in moderation and be sure to replenish fluids and to eat Kidney-energy-enriching herbs and foods afterward. Later in this season as we are ushered into winter, many people experience seasonal affective disorder (SAD). If you're like most people with SAD, your symptoms start in the fall and continue into the winter months, draining you of energy and making you feel depressed. While closeness and touch can certainly help lift your moods, you should not engage in sexual activity when you are feeling tired, depressed, or emotionally unsettled, as this too will only take from the very life essence you need to see you through this time. Be sure to engage in tenderness and loving acts without climaxing, as this will fortify your *Jing* without causing you to lose it.

The **winter** is the time to actively preserve your Kidney energy, which is stimulated by loving cuddling. The longer you cuddle and the more sexual sensation you experience, the better. However, men should refrain from ejaculating too often during this time of year as it will consume too much of the Kidney energy vital to ensuring your longevity and regulating your aging process. This really is the time of year for rekindling emotional ties and fortifying sexual energies, not depleting them.

Chinese medicine also teaches us that when sex is a purely physical act, energies are expended, whereas when deep emotions are involved, energies are actually exchanged and enhanced between the two parties. Lovemaking is therefore preferable to casual sex or masturbation anytime of year.

About Sleep Patterns by Season

Just as with exercise and sex, we all know that having enough tranquil sleep is vital to our health and to the image we project to the world. However, many people don't yet realize that what time you begin and end that period of sleep can be just as strong a factor in maintaining your overall health and beauty as how many hours of rest you get. As a general rule, you should rise and sleep in sync with the rhythms of the sun and the moon, which, of course, vary with the seasons. To make it easy for you, just remember that:

In the **spring, summer, and late summer,** you should go to bed later and rise earlier. These are the seasons when *Yang Qi* rises and grows stronger, and when the days are longer than the nights. Following these seasons' energy flow means getting less sleep at these times of year than at others.

In the **fall,** you should go to bed early and rise early. During this season, the days become shorter and the nights become longer. It is nature's way of telling us to sleep more so we are better prepared for the winter ahead.

In the **winter,** it is wisest to go to bed early and rise late. You want to conserve as much energy as you can in order to restore and revitalize the body's *Jing, Qi,* and *Spirit.*

Year-Round Sleep Tips

Of course, there is more to sleep than just when you arise and when you lay your head down to rest. The following tips will help you get a good night's sleep no matter what the season.

Head to the East to Sleep

According to Chinese medicine people should sleep with their head to the east, where the sun rises. Since the head is where all the *Yang* energy meets, it will be perfectly poised in this position to greet the early morning's growth energy.

Sleep on Your Side

Sleeping on your side keeps the airways open, leading to a deeper and more restful night's sleep. Chen Tuan, the Taoist Sleep Deity of the Song Dynasty, recommended sleeping on your left side while keeping your left leg and arm bent, your left hand touching your head, and your right leg straight while your right hand rests on the thigh of your right leg. If you really must sleep on your right side, assume the same pose while lying on the opposite side of your body.

This position creates a smooth energetic circuit that benefits the Heart, Liver, and brain—the organs that most inform restful sleep.

Keep the Lights Off

To keep from compromising the quality of your sleep, be sure to turn all the lights off in your room before bedtime.

It also helps to refrain from listening to loud music or watching action-packed television shows for at least an hour before turning in.

Soak Your Feet in Warm Water Before Sleep

Before you go to bed, preferably at 10:00 P.M., you should immerse your feet in warm water for approximately fifteen minutes. The water should be a slightly higher temperature than your body temperature to achieve the best results. This practice helps your Kidney *Yin* energy connect with your Heart *Yang* energy, and harmonizes both your Kidneys and Heart for a restful night's sleep.

Meditate Before You Sleep

Quiet generates *Yin* energy, and the stronger your *Yin* energy is, the sounder your sleep will be. For this reason, you should meditate for fifteen to thirty minutes before bedtime, focusing your mind on the here and now.

You should also sleep in a silent room. As much fun as pillow talk can be, remember that staying up to chat can consume vital life energy. Set the tone for a restful and restorative night's sleep by following these simple rules.

Keep Food and Beverages with Caffeine to a Minimum

The caffeine contained in coffee, tea, chocolate, and soda tends to excite the central nervous system, compromising the quality of your sleep. These stimulants increase the body's sympathetic and stress reactions, placing additional strain on the Liver and Gallbladder. For this reason you should limit food and drink with even the mildest levels of caffeine in the evenings, making sure that none are consumed after 12:00 P.M.

Sleep Well Clothed According to the Season

When people are asleep, they are not always well positioned to protect themselves from exposure to the Wind or Cold, especially during the spring and summer months when windows are open or air conditioners are on. Exposure to these elements during sleep can easily lead to headaches as well as shoulder and neck pain. To avoid these ailments and others, be sure to sleep with clothing and bedding that protect you from drafts.

Sleep During the Hours That Are Best for Your Body

Refer to the chart on page 23 to see what times of night your *Qi* is nurturing various organs. Bear in mind that the two most important times to rest for optimal health are:

From 11:00 P.M. to 3:00 A.M. These are the hours when the Liver and Gallbladder detoxify and recharge. These two organs are major players in the healthy functioning of your system during the daytime. Allowing this meridian the time it needs to rest and replenish is vital to healthy living.

From 11:00 A.M. to 1:00 P.M. These are the hours when the Heart is being replenished. Taking a nap for thirty to sixty minutes before 1:00 P.M. aids the body's recovery from everyday stresses, as does regularly being in bed before 11:00 P.M. each night.

WHAT TO DO IF YOUR SLEEP HOURS ARE IRREGULAR

I recognize that many of you are too busy to stick to the hours and sleep suggestions offered in this book. The hard-driving American lifestyle keeps the majority of us from getting the quality rest we need. Others of you may be unable to get enough sleep because you are night-shift workers. Over time, people with these reversed schedules tend to suffer the most. Their health and outer appearance show signs of how taxing working against your body clock can be. In fact, many of these folks suffer from a condition called shift work disorder. It is marked by a desire to nap during waking hours. Patients with this disorder have an uncontrollable urge to doze off, even in the midst of activities. They frequently experience impaired mental acuity, irritability, lower performance levels, and a proneness to accidents.

Whatever your reasons for staying up later than you should, the following precautions are offered to help you sleep better whenever you can. **"Getting your beauty rest" is not just an idle expression.** Sleep is among the most important factors in ensuring our health, well-being, and a perennially fresh face!

Nurture Your Heart Before You Sleep

Your Heart is not only in charge of your blood's circulation, but it is also the center of your consciousness and spirit. Even when you are asleep, your Heart is still working. For this reason you should eat a small amount of Heart-nurturing foods in the early evening to aid your sleep and the replenishment of your Heart's energy. Nourishing Heart foods include soups cooked with lotus seeds and *Lilium*. (*Lilium* is known as the daylily in the West and is not only edible, but incredibly tasty too.) Another nourishing Heart food is millet congee, which is essentially millet porridge. You can add spices and fruit such as dates, plums, and lychee to this congee for added flavor and texture.

Warm Your Tummy for Better Sleep

Stomach disturbances interrupt sleep all the time. Keeping your tummy warm can ensure a better night's sleep. Wear at least two layers of cotton clothing to bed, especially during the winter months when you will need to warm your Stomach. People who have frequent stomachaches can also add ground ginger or cinnamon to the lining of their covers to help alleviate their pain and treat the underlying cause.

Protect Your Gut When Staying Up Late

Staying up late can cause the dysfunction of your digestive system, resulting in acid reflux, indigestion, gastric ulcers, stomach pain, diarrhea, and/or constipation. When you have to stay up late, be sure to have a light snack between lunch and dinner, especially if you tend to eat dinner later than 8:00 P.M. You should avoid eating snacks two hours prior to bedtime as well.

Also avoid foods that are spicy and hard to digest, especially fermented foods, glutinous rice, sweets, and, of course, strong teas or coffees.

Don't forget to make an extra effort to increase your intake of fresh fruits and cooked vegetables too.

Protect Your Eyes When Staying Up Late

Staying up late may cause dry and achy eyes as well as blurred or weakened vision. When you have to stay up late, try to close your eyes for ten to fifteen minutes each hour. Massage the area around your eyes, and be sure to eat foods or take supplements that are rich in vitamins A and B.

Also eat plenty of leafy green vegetables such as spinach. Add yellow- and orange-colored vegetables such as carrots, squash, and grapefruit, and enjoy a variety of fish, including tuna, salmon, bass, and eel.

Protect Your Skin When Staying Up Late

Staying up late may cause skin to age faster, to become dull and dry. It can also cause dark circles or bags around the eyes, and increase wrinkles, sagging skin, acne, and freckles. When you have to stay up late, be sure to remove your makeup and supplement your diet with water and foods rich in collagens and vitamin C. You should also avoid salty, spicy, and greasy foods. Apply a facial mask and massage for ten to fifteen minutes.

Protect Your Immune System When Staying Up Late

Staying up late may cause compromised immune function, autonomous nervous system dysfunction, adrenal fatigue, colds, allergies, and digestive problems. When you have to stay up late, be sure to meditate for thirty minutes every day, focusing on life here and now, maintaining a happy mood and a peaceful mind, and remember to laugh and smile a lot throughout the day!

Also be sure to eat healthy proteins, vegetables, fruits, garlic, and a variety of grains. Avoid sweets. Take hot baths and exercise regularly.

Protect Your Brain When Staying Up Late

Staying up late may cause memory loss, poor concentration, forgetfulness, slow responses, headaches, insomnia, and an increased risk of dementia. If you must keep a late schedule, you should eat foods that are full of unsaturated fatty acids such as nuts, black sesame seeds, and olive oil. Avoid red meats, animal fats, and dairy. Also be sure to eat foods or take supplements with a full range of the B vitamins.

Protect Your Endocrine System When Staying Up Late

Staying up late can cause the deregulation of hormones in the body. It can also cause hyper- or hypothyroidism, decrease your libido, lead to infertility, obesity, endometriosis, breast disease, diabetes, prostate disease, acne, hair loss, and mood swings. If you have to stay up late, maintain your nutrition and energy levels with fresh fruits, vegetables, herbs, and supplements. Avoid sweets, and increase your daily physical exercise.

Include Foods in Your Diet That Help You Sleep Well

If you have trouble sleeping, be sure to work the following foods into your diet. They tend to help multiple organs at once so they can all coordinate to aid your sleep.

Avocado
Honey
Milk
Red Dates
Tofu/soybean
Turkey
Vinegar
Walnuts

Massage the Following Acupressure Points to Help You Sleep Better

An Mian is an acupoint that helps achieve peaceful sleep. It is located behind the ear below the base of the skull, as illustrated here.

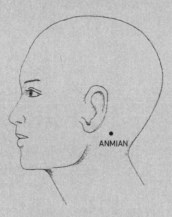

Bai Hui is the point located where the line from one ear tip to the other intersects with the midline of the head, as illustrated here.

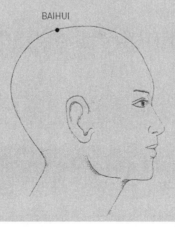

Shao Hai is located at the midpoint of the line connecting the medial end of the transverse cubital crease and the medial epicondyle of the humerus when the elbow is flexed, as illustrated here.

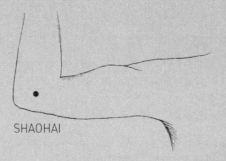

SHAOHAI

Shen Men can be found at the wrist crease located at the base of the pinky side of your palm, as illustrated here.

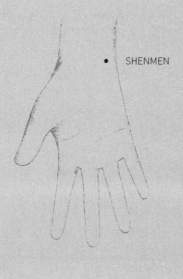

SHENMEN

Zhao Hai lies in the depression just below the tip of the medial malleolus, which is the bone that protrudes on the inside of your ankle, as illustrated here.

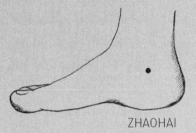

ZHAOHAI

Tai Chong is located on the dorsum of the foot in the depression at the junctions of the first and second metatarsal bones, as illustrated here.

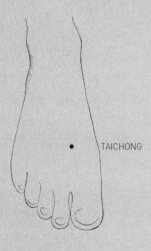

TAICHONG

PATIENT-TESTED TRUTHS

There are several examples of times when patients who have become better at-tuned to their body's energetic needs throughout the different seasons have made changes to their lifestyle that have yielded resoundingly positive results.

Fifty-year-old Moira came to me distraught because after so many years of daily jogging through all kinds of weather, her knees were failing her. She knew she needed to make a change, but she didn't know what sport could possibly elicit the same passion. Even before helping her figure that out, my immediate goal was to improve blood and Qi circulation to the well-worn area. Often, blockages, such as swelling and scar tissue from repeated trauma, and Blood Stagnation, from icing a painful joint too much, impede the flow of Qi to those joints and surrounding ligaments and tendons. Acupuncture clears the pathway for this healing energy. Moira's recovery was remarkably quick. After just a few sessions she was feeling active again. To steer her away from daily exercise that is as intensely repetitive as running, I encouraged her to rotate jogging with swimming. Swimming is a non-weight-bearing sport *and* its strokes can be varied to work different parts of the body. This ensured that she was no longer stressing the same joints and muscles over and over again. I also introduced her to qigong because this form of exercise can be conveniently done anywhere, anytime of the year, and it not only conditions the body, it is also known to boost alpha brain waves. The results of engaging in these different types of athletics that can be done with less stress year-round have been marvelous for her. She enjoys a relaxed mind frame while improving both her mental and physical agility. Moira is as happy with her new regimen as she is with the restored health of her knee. As a bonus, the increased circulation and the freedom from chronic pain have brightened her face, taking years off her appearance.

Forty-two-year-old Yvonne suffered from insomnia. She is a college professor who often stays up late grading student papers. Nothing she did could help her sleep straight through the night. With the help of some herbal remedies, acupunc-ture, a significant change to her seasonal diet, and a new bedtime schedule syn-chronized to seasonal light changes, she began enjoying the best sleep of her life.

Not only did her colleagues say that she looked younger, but the dean noticed her improved energies and mood. She was asked to speak about her experience in a class on natural health practices.

Lastly, twenty-eight-year-old June had been trying to get pregnant for more than three years. She and her husband, Kenny, had nearly exhausted fertility methods when they came to me to pursue acupuncture. Research shows that acupuncture increases the success rate of in vitro fertilization. It is believed that, based on a Chinese medicine assessment and diagnosis, the stimulation of certain trigger points on the body by acupuncture needles prompts the body to release select hormones and chemicals that can reduce pain, regulate the endocrine system, minimize inflammation, and calm the nervous system. Because I believe that stress reduction, nutritional support, and a healthier lifestyle can increase the chances of pregnancy, I began to take other steps as well to improve their chances of conception. After twelve acupuncture sessions, dietary changes to include season-appropriate foods that would best supplement the nutrient value of the endometrial lining, and the implementation of stress-reduction techniques and sexual practices, the couple now has a very happy little baby girl!

Norma's Musings on Surviving Long Winters

I enjoy designing for every season. At heart I'm really a warm-weather person. I'll take the sun and water any day. I feel like a flower blossoming in the summer months. I love to be outdoors and I especially love being at the beach. You can see that reflected in the collections I've designed over the years. Yet I know some people who are more invigorated by the chill of the winter. All I can think about whenever they want to be outdoors in twenty-degree weather is, *You've got to be kidding!* The winter is actually a very challenging season for me. I'm always trying to protect myself from the cold and darkness. It feels like nothing's living during that time. The days are short too so I find myself doing everything I can to adjust to the lack of light. I'm an early bird—I'm out by 5:30 in the morning on most days. In the hours between heading to the studio and arriving home again I often feel as if I've had no exposure to sunshine. We have skylights in the office but I'm still mostly surrounded by artificial light. I take vitamin D_3 to help, and I consciously eat foods that are going to make me feel better. But this year I have decided to close the office for a week in mid-February so those who work with me and celebrate Chinese New Year can do so with their families or go somewhere warm and bright to recharge. It's so important to have a healthy dose of natural light during this season even if you have to plan for it or head out of town to get it.

Just as Dr. Yang suggests, I also fortify my body during this time. I make a serious effort to eat foods that are compatible with my system. I am lactose intolerant, so I am constantly in search of options that contain calcium. I started drinking quinoa and hemp milks recently. It sounds bizarre, but I will frequently grind flax seeds up with one or the other. The combination contains a lot of valuable nutrients, proteins, and fibers that make me feel good. Even if you don't have a lactose issue, you may want to try it. I also challenge myself to avoid the holiday temptations of fruit and sweets. I get sick in a nanosecond if I have more sugar than my body can handle, so I avoid it. I do enjoy cacao, which is raw unprocessed chocolate naturally packed with antioxidants, essential vitamins, and minerals, in small bits. I also believe in eating foods that are in season, so in the winter I'm squash happy. I love all the different colors and flavors it comes in. I'm not a great cook, and I eat a lot of raw foods, but for heat and warmth I absolutely love all the variations of this vegetable, from pumpkin, butternut, acorn, and spaghetti squash to the more exotic red kuri squash. They are a great source of anti-inflammatory nutrients, including omega-3s and beta carotene, and they provide a real boost to your immune system so they are super helpful in staving off colds and the flu, among other illnesses. I put them in the oven and let them cook. Sometimes I let them get really soft and eat them like porridge for breakfast. Other times I make a soup from them. Some are sweet so I have them as a treat. If you cook them for a long time, they caramelize and taste great. And when you whip them up with flax seeds and nuts, they're *amazing*. You can't get better than that. I also eat raw vegetables cut up in a bowl with olive oil, lemon, and turmeric. It's a fantastic munchy snack loaded with great vitamins, and you can eat as much as you want. There's something about crunchy chewing that's really satisfying. The more you become attuned to your body and eat seasonal and wisely prepared foods, the more you will realize that there is a difference between cravings and really wanting the things that your body needs.

My other tip for surviving the winter is buying the best bed you can find. It doesn't have to be expensive, it just has to be right for you. Invest the time to find the perfect mattress. Lie down on the mattresses in the store and see how each one feels before making your purchase. You want one you can just sink into for hours on end while having support. Once you pick the one that provides the ideal retreat, you are set for even the harshest months. It will not only provide you with all the comfortable sleep you require, it will be the place where you and your significant other hang out, kiss, hug, and cuddle... and where the kids and the family pet can all nestle with you too. It's also where you can nap while reading a book or watching a movie. Napping is a luxury of mine in the winter. I am not someone who can thrive on just five hours of sleep a night. I need a solid six or seven hours, and if I happen to nap during the day in the winter too, then good for me. I know that my body needed the rest and that I gave it what it asked for.

Despite my dislike of the cold and darkness, it was these very conditions combined with my longing for a warm comfy bed while I was camping outdoors one evening that led me to design the sleeping bag coat—which is proof that if you really listen to your body's needs, you can innovate around any challenge the seasons present! And, of course, following Dr. Yang's suggestions will help see you through any other conditions you can't navigate that way.

12

Weighing In on Body Issues

A BALANCED APPROACH TO MANAGING DIET AND EXERCISE

There is no doubt that weight is an obsession for American women, but the truth is that it's an obsession for women everywhere. I have a friend who is involved in combating this issue globally and she tells me that it's universal and it's epidemic. Women in Brazil, India, and Afghanistan are worried about their weight, too. Cultural messaging, self-esteem, and the availability and understanding of healthy foods are all contributing factors. Women are in constant turmoil over knowing what they should eat, how much they should eat, and when they should eat. **Dr. Yang, what is the Chinese medicine perspective on weight and managing it healthfully? Is there some insight that can help us understand and deal with it better?**

You are right to raise this issue in a book where we are casting a different perspective on the relationship between health and beauty. In many ways, the subject of weight gets right to the heart of how classical Chinese medicine is extremely relevant today. There is too much unnecessary pain occurring in our culture and all around the world over body weight because we consistently fail to take a more balanced view of it. The emphasis is all too often placed on standards of appearance rather than health, when in fact, beauty is a result of good health. My study and practice of classical Chinese medicine tells me there is only one way to redirect the dialogue on weight, and that is to examine it on multiple levels—structural, biochemical, bioenergetic, emotional, and spiritual.

When a patient with a concern about their weight enters my office, I first look to see how healthy that patient is. That is more important to me than any number on a scale. There are certainly many overweight patients who are at risk for serious medical conditions such as heart disease, diabetes mellitus, high blood pressure, and cancer. But there are also patients considered to be "overweight" by societal norms who are very healthy.

The overweight person who is *healthy* must accept that they are constitutionally or prenatally different from others and they should continue doing all that they can to be the best version of that genetic disposition they can be. It is just a fact of life that some of us are born to weigh more or less than the person next to us.

Those who are overweight and *unhealthy* must realize that they too may be constitutionally or prenatally different, but that their postnatal choices are likely contributing to their weight as well. Greater understanding of their eating, exercise, and lifestyle habits and their emotions is in order to achieve better overall health and wellness.

By the way, I see just as many patients who by societal norms are considered "enviably thin" and they too must evaluate their prenatal disposition and postnatal choices.

Everyone should think about the practices we have been discussing so far in relation to their weight. Do you get enough nurturing sleep, or are your late hours compromising the ability of your Qi to refresh and replenish vital organs, including those involved in converting food to energy? Do you eat at the optimal times of day? Are you choosing the right foods for each season? Are they fresh and locally grown? Are you getting enough variety of foods? Are you living in the right climate? Is your environment too damp, thereby causing inflammation throughout your body? Or is it too hot, causing you to lose valuable Qi through constant perspiration? Are you exercising? Is the physical activity you're engaging in right for the time of year you are doing it? Do these activities energetically balance or hurt you? Are you using your sexual energies wisely? Are you worrying too much? Are you comfort eating—or not eating enough—in an effort to deal with stress, depression, or anxiety? Are you fighting undiagnosed chronic inflammation and/or infection?

Poor dietary and sleep patterns, the wrong choice or lack of exercise, your level of sexual activity, and your emotional state are just a few of the factors that may be compromising your efforts to reach or maintain a healthy weight. To get to the bottom of why you may be carrying so much weight, it is important to examine the potential structural causes first. I will always check to see if the patient has joint or muscle pain, inflammation, or arthritis and I will, of course, address those issues, whatever they may be, so we can be sure they are not limiting the patient's ability to exercise or their mobility in general.

Next, it's important to look at the potential biochemical causes.

Is the patient's metabolism slow? Are they experiencing hormonal problems? Do they have a sluggish thyroid? Or adrenal challenges? On top of that, I will check to see if the patient has any food sensitivities that may be putting a chemical stressor on the body, or if they have parasites or candida. If the gut is not functioning well, it can absorb things that are not meant to be absorbed, causing an immune reaction that results for many people in inflammation that adds on pounds.

Naturally, I would also look at the energetic piece of the puzzle—the part that modern medicine misses. The two organs most obviously involved in weight management are the Spleen and Stomach as they digest, absorb, and metabolize foods. Chinese medicine tells us that eating too many sweets, consuming too many carbs that turn into sugars, or simply ingesting large quantities of fatty and oily food can put a great strain on the Spleen. When you eat later than you should, you are also requiring your Spleen and Stomach to work overtime, expending more than their allotted energies and contributing to their burnout.

The Spleen is also, as you know, associated with the emotion of worry, so it is perfectly understandable that many of us eat in reaction to that stress. (It is also likely that the reverse is true too—we feel stress because of the way we eat!)

Less obvious players in your ability to manage your weight—though very important players—are the Liver and Gallbladder. Referring back to the Theory of Five Elements chart on page 72, you will note that the Liver and Gallbladder are associated with Wind energy. When these organs are functioning properly, they make sure everything in the body keeps moving. They specifically regulate the activities of your Spleen and Stomach. If, for any reason, there is a blockage in the Liver and Gallbladder, their *Qi* will stagnate and the functions of the Spleen and Stomach will be adversely affected too.

Now this is where the energetic and emotional components of weight management collide. One of the most common causes of *Qi* stagnation in the Liver and Gallbladder is anger. When this emotion, which is often associated with past trauma, festers there, it blocks the flow of *Qi* and the ability of other organs, including the Spleen and Stomach, to do what they need to do. While it has become a common dietary practice for people to detox their Liver from time to time, these detox programs only provide a biochemical cleanse. They do not clear your Liver of built-up or hard-to-remove emotional residue. Your Liver and Gallbladder will remain clogged if you do not *energetically* detox them as well. You have to release whatever prior experience causes you anger, hurt, or bitterness so you can resume proper functioning of your metabolism. You must also learn new coping skills so you don't repeat the same responses to hurt that caused the stagnation to begin with.

This is often why people who are truly committed in their mind to dieting cannot seem to remain committed in their day-to-day actions. Motivational speakers will tell you that when you put your mind to something, there isn't anything that you can't do. But they are only partially right. You actually have to put your head and heart on the same page as your gut before you can ask them to act in sync with one another. And even when you do that, you must realize that although the mind may be ready to move on from an offending experience, the other two may not be. If you cognitively think, *This is what I want to do*, but you're emotionally ambivalent about it and you're physically appalled by it, nothing is going to happen. You will procrastinate, or worse, sabotage your own efforts. I call this clash between conscious and unconscious behaviors "emotional allergies." Basically, whenever you react against what the mind wants you to do, you are reacting to the past. You can only exert the mind's will when the past event has been scrubbed energetically from your body, and the mind, body, and spirit are congruent once again. Acupuncture and the neuro-emotional techniques we will talk about in the next chapter can help!

The anger that messes with your Liver and Gallbladder and, in turn, with your whole metabolism, can stem from a wide range of past hurts. In some cases, the trauma can be physical or sexual in nature, so the body's response is to build walls of protection (i.e., layers of fat) around itself. Other times, the trauma results from bouts of real and genuine hunger. The body literally holds onto whatever food it receives for as long as it can. Still other times, the trauma can be verbal. Our society routinely engages in fat shaming on both an individual and broad-scale basis. Many patients *internalize* this kind of criticism, regardless of whether it's coming from people they know or from a total stranger.

If we believe that every cell has a mind (and why wouldn't we since scientists are able to clone a whole being from just one cell?), consider how those cells are apt to respond when they hear disparaging remarks.

Almost every negative emotion associated with your appearance has been affecting how you manage your weight, and life at large, consciously and mostly unconsciously. These emotions include anger, resentment, fear, dread, paralyzed will, grief, worry, low self-esteem, feeling stuck or vulnerable. In fact, negative thoughts and emotions can actually affect how our cells behave as much as positive thoughts do.

There was a most amazing doctor of alternative medicine in Japan named Masaru Emoto. In 1994 he began to study the effects of music—and ultimately, the effects of thoughts, words, and prayer—on the formation of untreated distilled water crystals. The water exposed to positive messages created beautiful geometrical crystals while that exposed to negative messages looked too sick and polluted to form crystals at all. Seventy percent of our own body consists of water. Seeing its clear and dramatic responses to thoughts and words in Dr. Emoto's experiments should remind us all to be kinder and gentler when talking to our body about any feature, not just fat. And we should be kinder and gentler when talking about other people's bodies as well, as these thoughts and words can truly shape who we become. To my mind this kind of physical response to positive and negative messaging speaks very well to the spiritual and emotional component of the whole weight equation.

All of this is to say that when you understand the many different factors that affect your weight, you can begin to correct any imbalances that may be causing you to be anything other than what your prenatal disposition suggests you should be. And more importantly you can put the emotional and societal stress around the issue behind you. It will no longer be the insurmountable object standing in your way. No one should obsess about weight. For that matter, no one should obsess about health either because the very act of obsessing creates obstacles to your health. It introduces worry, which, in turn, impacts your Spleen and Stomach. **Remember, weight is not an issue of how much you weigh; it is an issue of how healthy you are.** Accept yourself as you are and you will see how your body complies with your efforts to nurture it back to good health. Weight loss then becomes a byproduct of your mental, physical, and spiritual well-being.

EASY THINGS YOU CAN DO TO START ACHIEVING A HEALTHY WEIGHT NOW

Stand before a mirror and really look at yourself. Appreciate the attributes you like most about your body. Pay yourself a compliment. You must not only think it, you must say it aloud. Remember the effect kind words had on Masaru Emoto's crystals!

Carry a copy of the Seasonal Shopping List from chapter 11 with you at all times so you can be sure to buy and eat foods that are healthy for you year-round.

Commit to taking a twenty-minute walk each day after dinner or choose from any of the following physical activities, all of which are gentle on your joints: yoga, tai chi, or qigong. If you cannot tolerate weight-bearing sports, consider a water aerobics or water dance class.

PATIENT-TESTED TRUTHS

Twenty-eight-year-old Lena is five feet six inches tall and weighed 195 pounds at the time of her first visit with me. She had been experiencing heart palpitations and shortness of breath, so she had gone to see her cardiologist. After taking a battery of tests, that doctor gave Lena a clean bill of health. He told her that her Heart was perfectly sound. Lena suspected that the stress of planning for her wedding and of trying to lose thirty pounds before the big day was probably the culprit. What was causing her even more frustration was the fact that since she began her pre-wedding diet, she had gained seven pounds. She was actually putting on weight instead of taking it off! She came to me because she heard that acupuncture was effective in helping to achieve healthy weight loss. Although she may have been right about the reasons for the recent spike in weight, I looked at her complete health picture to be sure. She mentioned that she had struggled with weight her whole life so it was important for me to investigate further. What I found was that she had several food sensitivities from eating such a highly restrictive diet for so many years. The recent effort to scale back even more just exacerbated the problem. Her diet consisted of the same foods, albeit healthy ones, every day. In addition to acupuncture treatments, I desensitized her from any negative emotions associated with her weight and weight control, and I varied her diet, reintroducing a more healthy balance of foods, including meats, fish, vegetables, fruit, and grains, the latter of which were almost completely absent from her meal plan before! Her mom's kitchen had always been a carb-free zone so Lena almost never ate breads, pasta, rice, or even the healthiest of grains, such as quinoa. As Lena began losing weight, she decided to change the menu for the wedding to reflect her new eating practices. Exerting some control gave her a great feeling as she had been letting everyone else—from her well-meaning family and friends to the wedding planner—make too many decisions for her regarding her and her fiancé's big day as well as her life in general. Gone were the feelings of helplessness, frustration, and anger . . . and gone too was the weight. Lena lost twenty-five pounds in eight months and continues to be radiant and healthy long after the wedding.

Norma's Musings on the Definition of Beauty and on the Importance of Stopping Objectification

When I was in sixth grade there was a girl who I thought was absolutely beautiful. She had long blond hair and a delicate nose. But more important, she entered the classroom as if she owned it. The way she walked in seemed to just announce, *I am beautiful.* She really believed it, and in believing it she managed to convince me and everybody else of it as well. Of course, I had dark hair and a comparatively big nose, so I knew fitting that particular definition of pretty was not within reach for me. Instead I strove to be unique and interesting and smart. But that girl taught me an important lifelong lesson: the value and power of confidence. I decided to try a little experiment after observing her. I imitated her just to see how it felt, and sure enough it felt great. Projecting self-assurance really is attractive. In the end, I'm happy that I didn't feel pretty back then because that can make you not want to try as hard to be all the other things you can become. I had to stretch myself to try to be important and different and special in ways that mattered more than being pretty. And besides, pretty doesn't really even last that long. Which brings me to what I believe is the definition of true beauty: when a person has a powerful, moving, or compelling story, you naturally feel connected to them, and in that one-to-one connection lies a pure kind of beauty. When someone is animated while they are talking, they are alive—and there is nothing more beautiful than when life is present and revealing itself. The telling of an authentic story can captivate all of us. A photo of a woman tells us a lot about the surface image, but I may not care about her the way I care about someone who is telling her story. She becomes more beautiful and less the symbolic ideal of a woman. All women have the potential to be beautiful. The message that women of every shape, size, age, and difference should embrace is that in our authentic selves and life experience we are naturally beautiful. Confidence and self-esteem bolstered by a healthy lifestyle are the real definition of beauty. I love the experiments of Dr. Masaru Emoto that Dr. Yang described for us. They teach us not only to send ourselves affirming messages about our own beauty, but also to resist the other messages people send that can often interfere with our developing sense of self.

As many of you know, I am engaged in a campaign to stop objectification in all forms, but especially the objectification of women. I produced a short film called *Hey Baby* and I launched the website StopObjectification.com, both of which are intended to foster a real and honest dialogue about the problem as it exists in everyday life. It is clear to me that objectification limits, decreases, and in many cases, eliminates a woman's ability to reach her full potential, and that is an assault on our humanity in every possible way. It has a lasting impact on us emotionally, physically, and energetically insofar as it results in a life unfulfilled. While thankfully most of us will never experience the worst kind of objectification, which of course is enslavement, the sad truth is that every woman on the planet will experience some form of this degradation in her lifetime. Because it's such a universal problem, it has to be looked at seriously. Why is having a bad hair day or feeling a little fat powerful enough to take us down? This culturally and self-inflicted sabotage begins at a very early age when girls are first sent signals that they are either pretty or not. They soon begin to objectify themselves in an effort to get others to care for and love them as proof that they measure up. It is a cycle that affects generations of woman and really must be stopped. In addition to embracing good health and letting that be our body's primary guide to beauty; in addition to sending ourselves self-affirming messages and acting confidently in all that we do; and in addition to pursuing a path that invites us to be the best and most interesting people we can be; we need to talk about the accumulation of experiences that have caused our body and self-esteem issues in the first place. And we need to do it in a manner and forum so men can listen and hear. Objectification doesn't only take place on the street. It occurs in our homes, in all kinds of relationships, and in the office too. I believe that all men, but particularly the fathers of all the girls who have ever been objectified in this world, have a valuable role to play. If their daughters tell them what the experience of being objectified has done to them, these fathers will become advocates in the fight to stop objectification with an intensity and passion that has to make a difference. I'm convinced that when fathers actually feel the full weight of their daughters' emotions in their body and their soul, they will have a transference so profound that they will influence their sons and other young men to be aware and to stop the bad behavior when they encounter it. Powerful and well-known men with daughters need to come forward first to help build momentum. When hurt like this gets trapped inside the body, it only builds. It's gotten to the point where it is going to take summoning the full force of society to change this, so I encourage all women to do their part by telling the men in their lives how objectification really feels. I genuinely believe most men have no clue about what a toll it is taking on the women they love because we just don't talk about it. Talk to them openly and honestly. Have them visit StopObjectification.com with you to hear the meaningful stories that other women have already shared; then ask them to help in engender change too. It will do a world of good.

3

Your Mind, Heart, and Spirit

13

Feeling Beautiful

THE ROLE OF EMOTIONS IN OUR OVERALL HEALTH AND RADIANCE

We've all noticed at some point or another that when we're suffering emotional distress of any kind, it's easier to get sick. I'm amazed at how often people who have just experienced a bad breakup, the loss of a loved one, or the loss of a job end up in bed with a cold, the flu, or sometimes illnesses that are far worse. Even if you manage to avoid getting sick, you can't escape showing signs of how you're feeling on your face and in the way you carry yourself. While most of us just chalk this up to stress, Chinese medicine understands this phenomenon on a much deeper level. **Dr. Yang, would you please tell us more about how our emotions actually relate to our health and ultimately to our appearance?**

I will gladly talk about this connection because recognizing that emotional distress is often the underlying cause of illness and disease is one of the great distinctions of classical Chinese medicine. A true understanding of this phenomenon, as Norma calls it, can be one of the most powerful healing, wellness, and beauty tools to have at your disposal.

As mentioned in earlier chapters, the forefathers of classical Chinese medicine had the unique ability to envision all of the energies that fuel human existence. What they saw when they looked at our complete system was that emotions—*and thoughts*—are actually components of *Qi*. They are energies that run along the same meridians as the energies nurturing each of our primary organs. Very specific emotions run along very specific meridians, which is why it is said that anger is associated with the Liver; joy is associated with the Heart; worry is associated with the Spleen; grief is associated with the Lungs; and fear is associated with the Kidneys.

Since *Qi* circulates throughout our entire body, leaving nothing untouched from the deepest inner recesses to the surface of our skin, you can understand how traces of emotional *Qi* can be detected in the eyes, mouth, complexion, hair, weight, and posture of a person. That is why we often say such things as: "She can't hide her emotions," "He's wearing his heart on his sleeve," or "Her feelings are written all over her face." I not only see emotion in the visible expressions of my patients every day, I see them in total strangers as I walk down the street. I don't know these people, yet I can tell their emotional state. When people are happy, they have a glow about them. When they are worried, their brows furrow, their foreheads wrinkle, their lips tighten, and their jaws clench. When we don't attend to our feelings, the signs of aging become much more pronounced and noticeable.

But even before emotion becomes apparent on the outside, it affects our internal well-being. When we experience emotional distress of any kind, the energy that serves our primary organs can be heavily impacted. Look again at the Theory of Five Elements chart on page 72. Note that the *Qi* that is expressed as grief runs along the same meridian as the *Qi* that nurtures the Lungs. The *Qi* that expresses the cognitive functions of restraint and discipline also runs along that meridian. This is why when someone is mourning the loss of a loved one, they almost always develop a respiratory infection and find it difficult to hold a clear thought in their head while they are dealing with their sorrow. In this case, grief blocks the flow of Lung *Qi* and results in mucus buildup and congestion as well as an inability to think about anything other than one's loss. As Norma noted earlier, sadness or a sense of loss can and often does land us in bed with a cold, flu, or worse.

Emotional trauma can misdirect *Qi* and can also cause blockages. When that happens, all kinds of symptoms, in addition to the ones already mentioned, can occur. These symptoms range from headaches, skeletal and muscular pain, irritable bowels and bladder, menstrual cramps, PMS, insomnia, tremors, and high blood pressure to depression, mania, agitation, and anxiety.

While most people are able to push emotional pain out of their heads over time, the emotional energy from major life events often stays stored in their hearts and guts for years. If the emotional issue remains suppressed or unresolved, this energetic response can be reactivated by even slightly similar life events, developing into severe pain, organ dysfunction, or consequently into a tumor, blocked arteries, cancer, or any number of degenerative diseases.

Now you see how energetic therapies such as acupuncture and acupressure can help one deal with both physical and emotional issues simultaneously.

In some instances, when our body fails to let go of this residual energy, it can easily trigger the same emotional response under new and different circumstances, causing us to repeat behavioral patterns that just don't make any sense—even to ourselves.

This is why people tend to develop addictions and why they find it so overwhelmingly difficult to overcome them.

You will have to find a way to release this stored emotional energy in order to fully clear the channel and resume the balanced flow of all your *Qi*. There are several effective ways you can do this, some of which we'll talk about in a moment. But first we must address what I call *the myth of stress*.

Practitioners of modern medicine have been poking around the edges of the emotion issue for a long time, but they are still missing what is right in front of them.

Whenever a patient has a malady that can't quite be explained by the results of a structural or biochemical examination, many Western doctors will tell their patient that stress is to blame. But there really is no such thing as stress or stressful events. Stress is one's *reaction* to whatever is happening; it is *not* what is happening. **When modern medicine talks about stress, it talks about it as the cause, but stress is really the response to a deeper emotion.**

When a practitioner of Chinese medicine sees a patient who clearly has an energetic imbalance resulting in pain, other symptoms of a developing illness, or behavioral patterns they wish to correct, we try to assess what else may be going on in that patient's life. Very often we will discover that some underlying emotion is driving their condition.

In addition to using acupuncture to help clear the associated channels, many of my patients have also turned to meditation. Both the science and spiritual communities of our time agree that daily meditation offers psychological and physical healing, reduces stress, alleviates depression, lowers blood pressure, relieves chronic pain and anxiety, and actually has the potential to make you happier. There is no denying that this practice is useful. After all, it has been around for thousands of years! In fact, some scholars have traced meditation as far back as 14,000 B.C. To support their timeline, they point to images in the ancient cave paintings of Spain and France that actually depict early cave men and women in meditative poses. More proof that the ancients hold secrets to our health that are every bit as applicable today!

In addition to meditation, I have also successfully used a method called neuro-emotional technique (NET). This is a mind-body technique that finds and corrects the energetic imbalances related to any unresolved emotion in the body, which typically manifests as physical, emotional, or behavioral issues. NET is a tool that can help improve many physical and behavioral conditions. Bear in mind that it does not cure or heal the patient, but it does remove blocks to the natural flow of vital *Qi* in the body, allowing the body to repair itself.

NET is not part of classical Chinese medicine; however, it is a great example of the way the theories of Chinese medicine regarding the relationship of mind and body, organ energy and pulses, can be applied and validated through therapeutic techniques.

I usually begin the technique by asking patients to hold one of their arms out straight in front of them while I firmly push on it right above the wrist. If the patient's arm muscle is able to hold its position under the pressure I am exerting but becomes weakened under the same amount of pressure after I repeat this action with my other hand touching their forehead, then I know the energies in that muscle are clear and it is a good test muscle to work with. If there is no change of muscle strength before and after I touch the forehead, I know they are *not* yet physically and emotionally aligned or ready for the process to begin. If that is the case, a couple of deep breaths usually help get them aligned. I then proceed by asking the patient to make a statement regarding the issue they are grappling with. For instance, if a patient is trying to quit smoking because he clearly knows it is bad for his health, but every attempt he makes fails, I will ask him to say, "I am okay with giving up smoking this time." If his arm goes weak under the pressure of my hand as he is saying this, then I know that while his head thinks this goal is his wish, his heart feels ambivalent, and his body is absolutely not aligned with his thoughts. These three—the cognitive, the emotional, and the physical body—must all be on the same page for *Qi* to flow freely through us and to generate any lasting behavioral changes.

To help determine where the emotion preventing him from kicking his cigarette habit is lodged, I will ask him to repeat the same phrase while I reapply pressure to his extended arm and use my finger to press the pulse points on the wrists along each of the primary meridians. I will soon discover which pulse point, when blocked, actually helps him to be able to make the statement and still hold strength in his arm. That means I temporarily blocked the negative emotional energy that was preventing him from feeling and acting congruently with his intention. As we know, each pulse point connects with each primary meridian and each meridian connects with specific emotions. I therefore have identified the emotional *Qi* associated with the meridian keeping him from fulfilling his wish. If, for instance, it is discovered that the Spleen meridian is causing the challenge, then I will test him to see if the emotion of worry, to which the Spleen is sensitive, is to blame. If this is the case, his muscle strength at this point will get weaker, which will confirm that it is indeed the emotion of worry that is at the root of the problem.

Next we want to find out how the emotion of worry is involved by asking the patient to try to complete the sentence "I feel worried about quitting smoking because . . ." Then we go on to find out if there is an earlier life event that generated the emotion of worry when he made changes in his life or when he had to give up something he liked or enjoyed. The body holds amazing memories of such events, physically presenting evidence of these memories when we continue using muscle strength as a form of biofeedback. Often we discover that an earlier life experience that generated worry at the time is subsequently reactivated whenever the individual faces even remotely similar events. The patient has been resistant to quitting smoking until this point because each time he tried he subliminally recalled the experience of giving up something that served a need for him. To help him get past this emotional and behavioral blockage, we then ask him to create an energetic circuit by closing his eyes and holding his hand to his forehead and pressing the Spleen pulse point (the one associated with worry) while visualizing prior events that caused him to feel this way and triggered him to resume smoking every time he attempted to quit. The patient will be invited to work his way backward as far as he can until he remembers all of the inciting incidents and negative emotions related to giving up something he relied on in his life. He will be told to breathe in and out as deeply as he can while visualizing each memory and connecting with the associated emotions. This will help him expel the accumulated emotional *Qi* from his body until all emotional residue associated with the original event is cast out.

For instance, a thirty-two-year-old patient named Rob wanted to quit smoking. He had tried many times before with no success. I began an NET intervention much like the one just described. During the ten-minute session, he told me his wife was pregnant, so he didn't want his habit to affect her health or the health of their future child. When I initially asked him to state his intention, he said he wanted to "give up cigarettes for good," but his arm grew weak, indicating that his heart and gut felt differently. As the intervention progressed, we learned that he enjoyed smoking because it gave him a chance to be outdoors for a few minutes during work hours and to take his mind off the pressures of the day. But while my patient *consciously* associated his habit with this small pleasure, it was a bigger *unconscious* association that was preventing him from being able to quit. Rob's dad had a very high-profile and prestigious job and had similar expectations for Rob, which he made known from the time Rob was young. After a particularly bad confrontation over grades when he was seventeen, Rob took up smoking less as an act of defiance and more because it gave him a reason to hang outside between classes and occasionally during study hall with some of the other kids who weren't stressing out about grades all the time. Contending with the workload of taking all AP courses was tough enough, but dealing with his dad's demands only created more worry for him. Just talking about that time in his life made Rob want a cigarette. But using the NET technique, he effectively breathed out all of the residual anxiety that was blocking the energy required to get his mind, heart, and gut in sync. On the day of our session—the day he discovered he was still holding onto the anxiety associated with the performance expectations his father had placed on him years ago—Rob quit smoking. It has been three years and he hasn't been tempted once. He is a successful individual who has proven to himself that he can handle stress without the need for cigarettes. Now a simple walk around the block gives him the five-minute break that smoking used to, and his new habit is far better for his health and for the well-being of his family!

Even if you don't have a specific goal you wish to meet or ailment you wish to address, you can identify and resolve underlying emotional issues before they ever develop into something more by using this technique. A patient named Karina proves my point. She came to see me shortly before Christmas. I asked her what she was doing for the holidays, and she told me that she hadn't decided yet. She was ambivalent about going home but wasn't sure why. I decided to help her with her dilemma using NET. As I applied pressure to her extended arm, she literally could not hold her own statements. She wanted the words "I am okay to go home" to be true, but as she said them, her arm collapsed. I discovered that when I pressed on her Liver pulse point—and the Liver pulse point only—I was effectively blocking that reaction, and her arm was able to hold its strength. Since the Liver Meridian is associated with Anger Qi, I continued the test to find out whether it was her own anger or her sensitivity to someone else's anger toward her that was responsible for her ambivalence.

The response of her arm indicated that it was actually both. By continuing to use its strength as a form of biofeedback, we realized the person in mind was her mother's best friend for more than forty years. Karina began to describe what had happened during the previous year. She said that when her mother passed away, all she wanted from the home she had grown up in was the family dining table. This family friend offered to store it in her home while Karina made plans to have it shipped to her apartment several states away. When the table finally arrived, she saw that it was scratched and that there was a coffee cup stain where there hadn't been one before. Karina said she just lost it. She was so furious that she yelled at her mother's friend. This friend ultimately admitted that she had been less than careful with the table when it was in her possession, but she also told Karina that she resented her outburst. Everyone in Karina's family told her that she had overreacted to the whole situation and should never have been so outspoken with her mom's friend.

So the question, whenever we have what others may perceive to be a disproportionate reaction to something, is "What's the 'over' part in our overreaction?"

According to NET, the "over" part is always the part of you that is reacting to the *past*. Once you have successfully backtracked to the original event in your life that triggered the anger you've stored in your body, you can effectively release it and free yourself of the conflict between what you want to accomplish and what you actually do accomplish. This technique can take you as far back as to when you were conceived. The body's memory of the event will guide you to it. In Karina's case, we worked back to age six. "So what happened at age six?" I asked her. I had known Karina for a while, and in that time she had never spoken much about her personal life, but all of a sudden it seemed as if she couldn't stop talking about her mother's abusive behavior toward her since the time she was very young. In many ways, this is where analysis and NET differ—these kinds of details are unnecessary in this type of intervention. The point in NET is not talking about what happened; it is to feel it, connect with it, and get rid of it. So I showed Karina how to create the energetic circuit we discussed earlier. As she began to visualize the first occurrence, she clearly stimulated the emotional connection. She then began to breathe in and breathe out until both the feeling and picture of each occurrence dissipated. After that I tested her again to see if there was any other emotion involved. Naturally it was fear, so we returned her to age six and slowly helped her to breathe that emotion out as well. When we finally tested her to see if she was now more comfortable with her wish, it was clear that she was. This time, her arm stayed strong when she said she was okay to go home. She was surprised by how powerful the experience was. Later, after she had returned from her trip, she told me that it wasn't about going or not going; it was about her getting physically and emotionally congruent with her own will. Just as Rob and all the others who have used NET to resolve long-standing emotional issues did, Karina put her head, heart, and gut on the same page too.

One of the great things about neuro-emotional technique is how efficient it is. I have certainly seen other modalities help people. Psychoanalysis is among them. Although Freud was right about almost everything—about transference, countertransference, consciousness and unconsciousness, childhood experiences backing adult behaviors, and more, his technique of free association is too inefficient. It is like trying to find needles in a haystack. And even if you are able to find those "needles," threading them to help piece together the patches of your life presents another challenge. While talk therapy is useful in helping us recognize cognitive distortions and learn new coping skills, it does little to alleviate what people have experienced during traumatic events in their lives at the emotional and physical levels. Neuro-emotional technique only takes a few minutes to help identify the underlying cause for our most troublesome behaviors and illnesses. It immediately brings them to your consciousness and provides you with a way to get rid of them. You literally breathe them out. To me, NET is a wonderful complement to conventional psychotherapies. And more important, it is another validation of Chinese medicine theories, especially the theories regarding the mind and body connection.

I am simply embracing the timesaving ability NET provides. Emotions that remain unresolved disrupt and block valuable *Qi*, shaving years off our lives. The balance NET brings to us in such a short time frame is an incredible tool for restoring mental and physical health, and helping us make positive changes in our behavior to achieve our full potential in life.

I am grateful to Drs. Scott and Deb Walker and Dr. Daniel Monti, who integrate the best of Western and Eastern life sciences in creating and teaching the neuro-emotional technique. For people who want to learn more, you can visit www.netmindbody.com.

MORE WAYS YOU CAN KEEP YOUR EMOTIONAL QI HEALTHY

Once you have gotten in touch with your emotional energy through meditation, therapy, or prayer—or have cleared your channels of residual emotion through NET—it is important to keep in touch with that energy and to keep the channels unobstructed. You can begin by:

Adopting a new view of the world that generates less emotional stress even in the presence of adversarial situations and life events. When you look at the things that typically trigger stress or emotional upset for you in a new way, you will feel and react differently. A person who believes that all of his problems are other people's fault will feel very differently when he begins to assume his own share of the responsibility. The less emotional stress we feel, the less likely we are to develop the kind of long-lasting energetic blockage that unconsciously affects our behavior down the road.

Breathing deeply while placing your middle finger on the pulse points associated with the emotions you are experiencing whenever you have just had a major emotional reaction to an event.

The following walks you through the process step-by-step.

1. Identify a negative emotion that is associated with a current or past life event.

2. Press the middle finger of one hand on the pulse point that correlates with the organ and emotion you identified (see the figure below).

3. Cover your forehead with the palm of your other hand and call to mind snapshots you associate with the negative emotion.

4. Take a deep breath in and out for a few minutes until the emotion and the images dissipate.

5. Repeat these steps for any additional negative emotions you associate with the issue.

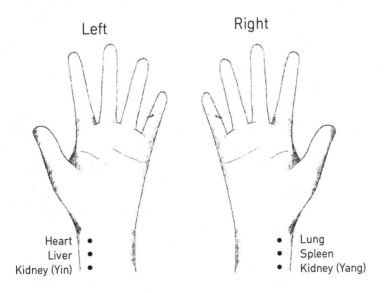

Of course, scheduling a few sessions with a certified NET practitioner (at www
.netmindbody.com) to periodically clear your neuro-emotional blockages would
optimize your health in all realms.

In time you will see that ridding yourself of years of emotional baggage is one of
the best beauty tips ever. Doing so will not only lift your mood, it will lift your spirit
and your face too.

Norma's Musings on the Power of Neuro-Emotional Technique

It's been interesting to read all the testimonials from Dr. Yang's patients
that have been included in each chapter so far. In this one, I must include
a testimonial or "patient-tested truth" of my own. When I first approached
Dr. Yang to learn more about how to improve my physical health and well-
being, I was interested in improving my emotional and spiritual well-being
too. I always try to be happy, centered, and satisfied with my life, but I want
to understand how to manifest even more love and joy. As Dr. Yang and I
became closer friends—and as we discussed the deep connections between
the health of the mind, body, and spirit—I began to share my hopes as well
as my fears on the subject of relationships. One day when I was visiting
Jefferson Hospital he and his colleague were eager to get me to try the
neuro-emotional technique he described in this chapter. They believed it
could help me unlock the reasons I was not yet dating the man of my dreams.
I was resistant at first to even trying the technique. I remember saying, "No,
no, no, I can't do this. I have to get back to the office now." But when I finally
gave in, I was really pleased that I had. Dr. Yang's colleague Dr. Dan Monti
took me back in time, mining the events of my life, and within two hours I
had arrived at the exact moment, time, and incident that set my fears in
motion. It was so fascinating to me. I'm a believer in sitting and talking and
having guidance, but psychoanalysis to me has flaws. The NET experience
was so effective I was able to unearth and release the thing I had buried so

deep in my unconscious mind—the thing I had allowed to own me for as long as it did—once and for all. I am happy to say that for the past four and a half years I have been enjoying the kind of relationship I have always wanted and deserved—a relationship with a truly kind, loving, and wonderful man.

Unfortunately we see examples every day of how emotions can cause energetic and behavioral blockages that keep us from living up to our truest potential, but what we don't get to see on a daily basis are the amazing effects that efficiently identifying and dealing with those emotions can have. I believe that this technique and others like it should be available to everyone so that this healing can happen much more frequently. I am incredibly grateful to the integrative centers that do offer this service to people and to the doctors who used it with me, making such a difference in my own life. Explore it for yourself and see what amazing things can happen.

14

Body and Soul

THE ROLE OF SPIRITUALITY IN WELLNESS AND BEAUTY

NK Dr. Yang, I know you ask your patients a series of questions to help them think more about how they perceive events in their lives. The answers to these questions should ideally enable them to understand their reactions and process their emotions in the most beneficial way possible. I also know that this is an integral part of your own spiritual philosophy. **Could you please share with our readers how, from your unique perspective, our spiritual life affects our health, beauty, and, in many ways, our active longevity?**

JY Yes, but first I wish to clarify that what I am about to say is strictly about getting in touch with your own spirituality. This is *not* a chapter about finding religion.

I truly believe that a healthy spirituality can help people let go of the kinds of past injuries and human attachments that thwart their energies and consistently get them into trouble. Throughout this book we have talked a lot about how you must be healthy to radiate visible and enduring beauty. This includes cultivating spiritual health, too, because if we are not spiritually healthy, we're not going to be emotionally healthy; if we're not emotionally healthy, we're not going to be socially and behaviorally healthy; if we're not socially and behaviorally healthy, we're not going to be biologically or physically healthy. And without this kind of comprehensive health we can't possibly attain the countenance, beauty, or vitality we seek. *All* aspects of our health must be nurtured for us to reach this goal.

I understand that there are many people who have no religious affiliations; however, *everyone* has to think from time to time about his or her personal answers to some very primary questions. Those answers may evolve as time goes by and as one's living experience continues. When these answers do evolve, they more or less reflect our spiritual growth. People's spirituality is constantly tested, challenged, redefined until the very end of their lives. Often, we as a species wonder if we are primarily human beings having a spiritual experience, or primarily spiritual beings having a human experience?

The following are five major questions that were listed in a medical textbook called *Current Diagnosis and Treatment*. I read it when I was taking my medical license exam in the United States. In this book, the medical model was redefined as a bio-social-psycho-spiritual model. I found it amazing that modern medical authors are recognizing the same level of complexities in human health that physicians who created Chinese medicine have for centuries. These are questions that you too can ask yourself now—and again periodically as you progress through life. Your answers will help define your spirituality, no matter what those answers are. I invite you to take some time and really think about them.

1. What is the meaning and purpose of your life?
2. What is your relationship with the people you encounter and the universe you live in?
3. Is there an existence of higher power(s)? If yes, what is your relationship to the higher power(s)?
4. Are there past lives, future lives, or after lives?
5. What do hardship, tribulation, birth, aging, illness, and death mean to you?

Life is really a very simple process: we come into it naked and crying, and we leave it naked and sleeping. In between, under normal circumstances, we burn all of our life energy by consciously or unconsciously reacting to the way we answer the preceding questions.

If, when contemplating the first question, "What is the meaning and purpose of your life?" someone answered, "It is to be as happy as I can be," it is conceivable that this person could turn to drugs for the initial pleasures they provide. If this person said, "It is to be as healthy as I can be," he or she could possibly become overzealous, taking tons of supplements and seeing so many doctors to be sure they are in peak physical condition that they ultimately become a hypochondriac. If this person said, "It is to be as rich as I can be," they could become a gambler, taking unnecessary risks to ensure their wealth. At times they might succeed; at other times they might fail. If the meaning of their life were defined in any of these ways, their emotions would be ruled by whether they achieved these states or not.

But what if the meaning of life is to learn from whatever life presents to us? **Wouldn't the perception of our experiences—and the experiences themselves—be very different?** We would try to learn when we lost money *and* when we made it; we would try to learn when we are well *and* when we're sick; we would try to learn when we're happy *and* when we're not. These are much more even-keeled reactions to life than the earlier set of perceptions and responses, to say the least.

Let's imagine for a moment that the meaning and purpose of your life is to return to where your meaning, purpose, and life was actually created. That your life was conceived in a higher place than earth and that you were just dropped into the human form with the expectation that you find your way back to this beautiful place of origin. How do you suppose you do that? One possible way my own spiritual teacher suggests is to cultivate your mind and body to their original pure state. If you want to go back to the beautiful place, you must first meet the requirement of admission physically and mentally. You need to adopt the mind-set and bodily characteristics of those dwelling in that place. If you're not mentally and physically prepared to be at a certain level, then you can't be there. You won't even want to be there because subconsciously and perhaps even consciously, you know you can't survive there. So how do you get to the point where you're ready, able, and willing to get there?

It comes with preparation and practice. In your lifetime here on earth and in this body, you will be presented with various opportunities to learn how to cultivate your life. The choices have to be made by you with the sole motivation to cultivate your body, mind, and spirit to be a better person. When you decide to pursue a life cultivation, in all life events—many of which involve pain and loss while others involve pleasure and gain—you will make choices that people up in the beautiful place would make. You will do so without any prior knowledge of what the true answer to those challenges might be. The more you make choices in this manner, the closer you will get to your place of origin. That is the meaning and purpose of your life: to take every opportunity to improve your mind and your heart, particularly in situations where anger or hurt would have otherwise been your first response. Everything that happens would be a good chance for you to respond in a way that enables you to ascend to the level you are hoping to get back to. **This belief system is the foundation of the whole Chinese culture and of Chinese medicine.** To be quite honest, it was not until I fully embraced this spiritual reality that so many of the intricacies of classical Chinese medicine I had been learning all my life became crystal clear to me.

When I began to believe that my soul will never die and that my life will never vanish but will reincarnate, I felt a great sense of hope and the urge to take better care of my life now. I also felt less sadness and pain when facing the loss of a friend, patient, or a loved one in my life.

When I started believing that one's soul has come a long way and has had many lives before this one, I felt less puzzled by the diversity of the world and the life experiences of people. Instead of reacting negatively in situations where I suffer loss, humiliation, or pain, I pause and respond more calmly. I also watch myself more closely to be sure that I do not abuse or take for granted what I have in life. When you put your own life in the spectrum of the universe, one lifetime is like one day—or even less time than that.

If you were to erase your memory of yesterday, everything happening today would be puzzling to you. Of course, we have no control over what might have happened in our past lives, but we do have control over what we chose to do in this lifetime, so our future or our next life will be better and brighter.

With my new knowledge, I began to understand the real meaning of the saying "What goes around comes around." Everything we do creates eternal energies that we call karma, which must be balanced. The universe has an incredible way of keeping this order. Without such balance we wouldn't have the seasons or a predictable sunrise and sunset. If you did something to another person, it has to be evened out with or without your agreement or intention. In Chinese philosophy, a gain can actually be a loss and a loss can actually be a gain. I know the assessment from a human perspective can be the opposite of the divine perspective. Chinese philosophy calls good karma *De* and bad karma *Yeli*.

When the scholar Lao Tzu wrote the book *Tao Te Ching*, he explained the physics of this energy. He defined *Tao* as the way and *De* as the substance we're talking about—this high-level energy that constitutes one's personal character and strength. *De* and *Yeli* are basically the good and bad energy that determine your future. They go with you life after life. *De* develops from a deed that is kind, honest, and selfless. *Yeli* accumulates by the behavior that is the opposite. This great teacher, Lao Tzu, says it is good to be dull instead of sharp, meaning one shouldn't care about one's personal interests or about trying to get the upper hand. Buddha says that being taken advantage of is your fortune. Jesus says to turn the other cheek when we are affronted. What they are all encouraging is the cultivation of *De*—the cultivation of a higher-power health and well-being.

We are afforded choices every day to help us attain the virtue of good health and fortune in this life and attain entry into a better place for the next life. Of course, when people first begin to grasp this concept they ask, "Does this mean that you should not seek medical attention when it is needed?" My reply is always, "No, it simply means that medical practitioners can help you to a point by attending to your structural, biochemical, and bioenergetic needs, but cultivating the higher-power health we are talking about is between you and the universe. The way you care for your body even more lovingly is to care for your spirit, too." In the end, how we perceive and respond to life events can determine—for better or for worse—our emotional experience, and in turn, our actions, health, wellness, and beauty in this life and certainly in the next.

When we cultivate this kind of complete health, our bodies truly reflect it. Spiritual energy is a healing and rejuvenating energy. We can now understand more fully how and why we appreciate so many different kinds of beauty. Beauty is less about what specific mix of features one possesses and more about how much inner health those features reveal. The same can be said of the most beautiful gardens, which grow from the most balanced, fertile soil.

Because spiritual energy, fortitude, and commitment have the power to change one on a molecular level—opening up the acupuncture points and meridians to greater reception of these qualities—they can also help us conquer what we perceive as disease or what is really the limitations of the body as we know it in this dimension. Theoretically speaking, spirituality is a type of energy—a much higher energy than all the other energies in our bodies. The *Qi* is, in effect, *mortal energy*, whereas the spirit is *immortal energy*.

Cultivating life by enhancing one's spirituality is, in a way, taking a giant step toward ensuring eternal beauty.

A RECAP OF WHAT YOU CAN DO TO CULTIVATE SPIRITUAL HEALTH AND WELL-BEING

Detox or cleanse your body of any residual emotions that can cause blockages or the repetition of damaging behaviors by using the NET methods described in this chapter or working with an NET expert or facilitator near you.

Pursue acupuncture treatments and/or massage your acupressure points to keep your energy channels clear of future blockages.

Begin a daily meditation practice for the same reason.

Maintain an exercise regimen involving qigong, tai chi, yoga, meditation, or
any other form of exercise that encourages the free flow of *Qi* without
stressing or damaging muscles and ligaments with repetitive motions. These
practices originate from life-cultivation systems known as *Xiu Lian*—the
more traditional and widely known of these include the Tao and Buddhist
practices.

Rethink and refine your responses to stressful events so you can rid yourself of
negative karma; augment your *De*, virtue, or positive karma; and generally
ready yourself for a higher-power existence.

Cultivate spiritual, physical, mental, emotional, and energetic health every
day. I personally benefit from the teachings of an original and authentic
life-cultivation system known as Falun Dafa—a system intended for people
living today (www.falundafa.org). In fact, I drew upon its wisdom to write this
chapter. The system involves practicing truth, compassion, and forbearance
at all times. It teaches the most complete and original qigong and meditation
techniques. People in the past have missed precious opportunities to study
and practice with the great teachers of their time. I hope people do not miss
the opportunity that is before us now.

Norma's Musings on Spirituality

Because self-examination can be very empowering, I've taken the time to
answer the questions Dr. Yang asked earlier in this chapter. I imagine all of
our responses will be deeply individual (which is perfectly in keeping with
classical Chinese medicine and with the true notion of beauty). Here are the
reflections these questions prompted for me.

1. What is the meaning and purpose of your life?
I don't think there is only one meaning or purpose to life, but the purpose
I have spent pursuing most publically is the goal of empowering women.

As a fashion designer I know there is a strong connection between what a woman wears and how she feels about her body. I have aimed to design clothes and to make health, beauty, and wellness available to women to nurture, embolden, fortify, and inspire them. And of course, my campaign to stop objectification is intended to do the same on an even deeper level. In my mind, an empowered woman is an invincible woman. And an invincible woman can do anything.

2. What is your relationship with the people you encounter and the universe you live in? Do you feel you've subconsciously invited certain people into your life?

The older I get, the more confident I am, so when I want to meet someone, yes, I definitely set out to find them and introduce myself. It's how I met Dr. Yang. I knew I wanted to talk with someone who had done non-surgical face-lifts successfully in the past, so I pursued that person and found this amazing authority in the process. Whenever I think there is someone who would be fascinating to meet, I get in touch with them and ask them, "Do you want to go to lunch?" In fact, I do this all the time.

Once my team and I were in the middle of developing a project. We were looking online for a neon display sign. While I was Googling various suppliers of neon products, I came across something called *Neon Animation*, which was incredible. It was this beautiful animated film about women. I turned to my assistant and immediately said, "I have to meet this guy, whoever he is. I have to talk with him—I'm so impressed with his work." So I reached out and made an appointment to see him. His name is Jack Feldman and he's this great guy—a wonderful character and person. We ended up spending such quality time together working on two films that were so fulfilling. Then we each went off again to do our own separate things. It was so special to have this fantastic creative bond and history together even if it was only for a specific amount of time, which brings me to another philosophy I subscribe to about people and the time we spend with them. More and more I believe that there is a certain amount of time we're supposed to share with those who come into our lives. It can be as short as a single meeting or it can last a lifetime. Some people are with us for a while and then they get married and move to a far-off city. Other people pass away and we not only feel their loss, we also feel the loss of some of our own energy—the shared energy that left with them. There are still other people who are meant to be with us for the long haul. There is a woman in my office who has worked with me for forty-six years. We met when she was eighteen years old. Neither of us would have guessed we'd be in each other's lives for nearly five decades. And not only do I believe we are we meant to be with people for a certain amount of time, but I also believe our relationships are meant to have a certain degree of intensity too, which can change over time. This is why when a parent dies, the separation and loss you feel if it happens when you are forty-eight years old is very different than what you might feel if it happens when you are twelve or eighteen. The comings and goings of people in our lives are meant to help shape us. They can be complicated and traumatic, as in the case of a young girl's first heartbreak or marital divorce. But each adds character-building experience to our life. And when we are having experiences, we are living and growing; when we're living and growing, we're alive; and when we're alive, we're infinitely more beautiful than when we're static and not growing and flourishing.

3. Is there an existence of higher power(s)? If yes, what is your relationship to the higher power(s)?

I consider myself very religious—I believe there is a higher power. *However, my religious belief is that this higher power resides within us.* To me it's a question of how godlike we can develop ourselves to be. I do believe there's this inspiration that makes us strive to achieve the ultimate behavior and the ultimate life. This is part of the process of spiritual growth we're meant to experience in this lifetime. But the power to do this has to be within us. If it's not our individual behavior that's godlike, where else is this power going to come from? How else is it going to manifest?

4. Are there past lives, future lives, or after lives?

I really believe that we're influenced by a very deep memory. I think it's not only the memory of our childhood and the things that have happened in this lifetime, but it is a memory that goes beyond that. As support for this theory, there are times when we think about things that are very disconnected from anything else in our lives—times when thoughts pop into our minds or things happen that we can't explain because they have no connection to our current life experiences. I think that children may have a clearer picture of those distant memories than we do as we get older, but that past-life memory stays with us as a spirit or energy throughout all our time. I totally believe that each life presents another evolution of that spirit—another opportunity to become closer to that godlike ideal. I think we are always given another chance to do it better and to get closer to a godlike behavior, philosophy, and existence. So yes, I believe we all carry a memory of the past, a sense of why we're here now, and what our purpose is in relation to previous efforts. As for the future, I believe that what happens then is largely the result of how well we do this time around.

5. What do hardship, tribulation, birth, aging, illness, and death mean to you?

I view hardship as a part of life, just as joy, happiness, birth, and their counterparts are. I don't think life can exist without it. It is part of the total experience. Periods of joy alternate with periods of hardship. Neither are going to last forever. It goes back to my answer in the previous question. How we deal with these experiences, what we learn from them, how we get through them is very telling about how evolved we've become and how well we're doing in this present life experience.

15

Being at One with Yourself

REDEFINING INTEGRATIVE MEDICINE

NK Much like I am, many people today are seeking therapies that are not offered by conventional doctors—therapies that tend to be natural, noninvasive, safer, and preventive and that address the whole person and the underlying causes of their chronic illness. What confuses so many people though are the various terms flying around, including alternative and complementary medicine, integrative medicine, functional medicine, and holistic medicine, to name a few. **Dr. Yang, you practice integrative medicine and psychiatry: How would you like our readers (who have already ventured toward a new way of thinking about modern medicine with us) to understand the term *integrative health* as they move forward in their health and beauty journey?**

JY Ah yes. This is a term that on the one hand can be incredibly misconstrued, or on the other, can help crystallize everything for us.

By now, however, those of you reading this book know the real meaning: When you care for each facet of your health completely and in tandem with the others, they work together in miraculous ways, bringing about truly lasting vitality inside and out. You understand that the brain is not the leader of all things. There is a balance of power within the human body, spirit, and consciousness that must be sustained for us all to endure and thrive. You know that human beings exist at the structural, biochemical, bioenergetic, and soul levels and that each depends on the other to help us remain alive and well. The codependence or cofunctionality of these energetic levels affects us physically, behaviorally, socially, emotionally, financially, and spiritually. Thus you also know there is no better way to care for yourself than by attending to *every* one of these four levels of our lives. **This is what we mean when we talk about integrative health.**

Integrative medicine in the West frequently means borrowing from the best practices of different cultures, as I hope more Western doctors will do with the teachings of classical Chinese medicine. But from the perspective of Chinese medicine, this term really means integrating the care of one's physiological, psychological, and spiritual health. Your overall wellness and beauty are contingent on *all* of your energies and biochemistry operating in balanced harmony with one another.

At its core, integrative medicine assesses and cares about a person at the structural, biochemical, energetic, and soul levels, utilizing the best tools we have to meet a person's needs fully. As a result, integrative medicine helps improve one's life in every way and all at the same time. It would be great if in the near future we no longer needed to use the term *integrative medicine,* because by its very definition it is what *all* good medicine should be. In fact, it is what every department of medicine in the world should be practicing!

Now that you have this understanding, it is my hope that whenever you wish to improve some aspect of your health or are pursuing a treatment for a specific ailment or disease, you will consider and choose therapies that address the needs of your whole being. Acupuncture, acupressure, herbal remedies, moxibustion, cupping, *tui na, gua sha,* and neuro-emotional technique, as discussed throughout this book, are all effective treatment modalities. So too are improved dietary, sleep, and exercise practices, the latter of which include qigong, tai chi, yoga, and meditation and their origins: life cultivation. When working with the right practitioner you can use these modalities alone, or they can be used to complement treatment being administered by your conventional medicine doctors.

I also hope that you will consider the interconnectivity of your energies when taking various supplements and medications. There are certainly times when these remedies are necessary, but there are also times when greater discretion and alternative care is in order. As you have read, despite the fact that each of us has a general energetic constitution, our energy is dynamic. It is constantly changing with the influence of external elements and pathogens. The broad claim that one type of vitamin, mineral, or herbal remedy is good for preventing or treating a specific condition in all people fails to recognize both the individuality and the dynamic nature of our bodies and their needs, our energies and what is required to balance them. Taking a daily dose of anything without proper assessment, follow-up, and modification by experienced professionals to hedge against some potential condition you may never develop could have other more serious consequences than the feared condition you are trying to preempt.

The long list of possible side effects from prescription drugs that many pharmaceutical companies now routinely make known to the public is also an indication of how different each of our responses can be. Just as is true of vitamins, our reaction to certain medications can be more serious than the conditions the medications were developed to address. According to the Food and Drug Administration, adversarial drug reactions are the fourth leading cause of death in the United States, costing over 100,000 lives annually. Then, of course, there is the added concern that many supplements and medications are designed to simply treat symptoms, not their underlying causes.

It is equally important to think about the effect on human energy that surgeries often have. Whether you elect to have surgery, as in the case of cosmetic surgery; are required to have surgery, as a possible lifesaving measure; or do so for any number of other reasons in between, recognize that invasive procedures can upset the balance of your energies because valuable Qi frequently escapes during such procedures. All nonessential surgery should be carefully evaluated. Be aware too that throughout the United States, surgeons operate on wrong body parts forty times a week. On some deep level Norma understood this when she sought my help in giving her an acupuncture face-lift in lieu of a surgical one.

Always make it a point to research any condition that calls for surgery, and investigate the Chinese medicine perspective on it too. Meet with a Chinese medicine practitioner to explore all the potential consequences such a treatment would have on your *Qi* and the organs running along the same meridian as the organ or feature being operated on. And discuss potential alternatives together as well. Invite your practitioner to talk with your surgeon so that if an operation or procedure is necessary, he or she can help complement your surgeon's work and speed your recovery along by fortifying your *Postnatal Qi* with acupuncture, herbs, dietary changes, and the many other remedies that may apply. Allow classical Chinese medicine to help make you as strong for the healing process as you can possibly be. In China, it is routinely used to refresh and revitalize women both before and after childbirth, and especially if the baby has been delivered via Cesarean section. The special wellness program women embark upon at this time is designed to help restore the *Qi* they lost in the birthing process. A wellness program can be also customized for you in advance of and in the aftermath of any type of surgery you may need.

People in the United States spend more on health care than people in any other country in the world, yet Americans' health status is the worst in comparison to that of citizens in eleven other developed nations and in a growing number of developing countries as well. We suffer more chronic illness and we die earlier too. People may wonder why, but if you pause to think about it, you will begin to see that the majority of our health care system exists *not* to keep us healthy, but to manage our chronic illness and deal with crisis. The tools U.S. doctors use most often include medications and surgeries that are also the tools health insurance companies will pay for. It is deceiving to call the services these companies provide "health insurance" when in reality what they offer is "sickness and crisis insurance." We need to stop thinking that all doctors, hospitals, medications, and procedures are taking care of our health because many are not. It is our responsibility to invest in and take care of our own health. I believe the only way to solve America's health-care crisis and to transform our *sickness-care system* into a true *health-care system* is by encouraging more people to adopt an integrative medicine approach. If you don't begin now, your health will decline and the first visible signs will be when your beauty and vitality disappear too.

Avoiding the need for medicine or surgery in the future—basically remaining healthy, alive, and vibrant—involves an **integrative approach** to balancing your energies every day. In many ways it's the ultimate preventive care. Each evening before you go to bed, ask yourself the following questions. Doing this will condition you to act with renewed awareness of your health and beauty goals as you go about your business the following day.

DAILY CHECKLIST FOR PREVENTIVE CARE

As you wind down for the night, ask yourself:

1. What did I do for myself structurally today? More specifically, what did I do for my muscles, bones, face, skin, and hair?
2. What did I do for myself biochemically? Did I eat enough nutrient-rich foods and drink enough water?
3. What did I do for myself energetically? Did I meditate, exercise, do qigong, acupuncture, or acupressure?
4. What did I do spiritually for this lifetime and the lifetime after that? Did I reflect on my actions, meditate, and extend honesty, compassion, patience and forbearance toward others and myself today?

I asked Norma to share her answers to these questions with us because she is always thinking of new, organic, and authentic ways to incorporate spiritual, physical, and mental health in her life and because so many of us recognize that she emanates genuine beauty in doing so. Here's what she said.

Norma's Musings on Everyday Practices

1. What did I do for myself structurally today?

I exercised at 4:30 this afternoon as I do every day. That is the time that's optimal for my body to exercise. I do an hour class a day and sometimes more. I love classes because when you're in a whole group, you're less likely to slack off. It's very efficient. I really think making sure you do some kind of exercise is more important than how long you work out or even what that exercise entails.

There are other things I did that are just part of my daily routine. For instance, when I took a shower this morning, I really let the steam and heat kind of loosen up my muscles as I did a round of stretching. We also have a bar in the elevator of my company building where we hang clothes as they are transferred from one floor to the next. I lift and hang from that bar every time I take the elevator. I find that it's a really good stretch and release for the spine. I take the stairs a lot throughout the day too because it's fast and easy and because moving around also energizes me. Twyla Tharp, who is a brilliantly talented friend of mine, appeared on a panel with me at the Museum of Modern Art and spoke about all the benefits of movement for your health. It's important for us to stay in motion throughout the day. Dr. Yang says that too. You can't sit and be sedentary. It's the worst thing for you. Movement keeps the blood flowing, the brain active, and the body alive. A lot of people are beginning to work at standing desks to avoid sitting for long periods of time. Other people have treadmill desks. I think there is something to this trend because it makes sure that both your physical and mental energies remain active. I'm fortunate because the fashion industry is a very physical business. I am always on my feet working in the sample room, moving racks of clothes around, or running up and down between the five floors of my building, so I don't have to make a conscious effort to get up and circulate. But if you are in a different line of work and find you are in meetings or at your desk all day, you must make the time to get the energy and blood flowing at regular intervals throughout the day and evening. So yes, I did that too. I definitely moved around a lot and kept the blood flowing.

2. What did I do for myself biochemically?
I drank a lot of water today. It's really important to remain hydrated. I also drank green tea. As we all know, it's loaded with antioxidants and reduces free radicals in our body, so our cells get an added level of protection that keeps them from aging. I also had a mixed greens salad with poached salmon drizzled with extra virgin olive oil for lunch. These foods are high in balanced and healthy fatty acids, which are also believed to extend our life expectancy.

3. What did I do for myself energetically?
I sought out silence today. As I mentioned earlier, I enjoy and need quiet time. Many people turn on the TV or play music the minute they get home, but I enjoy sitting in solitude with no other distractions for a few minutes. Silence for me is a form of meditation; it is a form of prayer. I believe in prayer, but my preferred prayer is more of a conversation. In any event, it has to take place in silence. Even if you do nothing more than sit in a chair and close your eyes, if you do it in silence, that to me is a meditation of sorts. So today I enjoyed a few moments of planned peace. I also had my weekly acupuncture session with Dr. Yang, which always puts me into a deeply relaxed state. After that, I felt energized, and my face was notably glowing.

4. What did I do spiritually for this lifetime and the lifetime after that?
I expressed love to the people I care about and found ways to be of service to them ... and I wrote these thoughts down in the hope that my practices might benefit others the way they've benefited me.

So, dear reader, I'm curious—what would your answers to these questions be today? What might they be six months or a year from now? How much health and vitality will be restored in that time if you follow our suggestions, monitor your energetic constitution, and reflect on these questions regularly? How many years will you have added to your life? And how many years will you have taken off your visible appearance? I hope we have inspired more than your curiosity with this book. I hope we have stoked your will and your energy to take the kinds of actions that benefit your *whole* body; to make the kinds of changes that bring you complete health, beauty, peace, and longevity; and to adopt a mind frame that allows you to face forward with true confidence. Lasting beauty really is yours to have with these coordinated efforts and time-tested methods.

Acknowledgments

This book has been a long time in the making. I wish to thank my loving family, especially my wife, Lan, and son, Kevin, who gave me unconditional support in this process, and of course my father, who introduced me to the ancient practices that led to my continuing love of healing and who bought me a radio to help me learn English when I was a kid. Many thanks as well to my colleagues at the Tao Institute of Mind and Body Medicine and Thomas Jefferson University Hospital, particularly Dr. Dan Monti, who is a great mentor and friend I can always count on for help. Much gratitude also goes to Norma Kamali, whose support and encouragement led me to actually write this book. I also wish to thank my agent, Alan Morell, for his wise and consistent counsel; my dedicated writing collaborator, Hope Innelli, whose skills added so much to this project; artist Naomi Sun for her fine renderings; Dr. Qi Wang for permission to use his invaluable questionnaire on physical constitution; and the incredibly professional, creative, and talented team at Harper-Collins Publishers, including Lisa Sharkey, Daniella Valladares, Paige Hazzan, Molly Waxman, Lauren Jackson, Leah Carlson-Stanisic, Andrew DiCecco, and Jeanie Lee. The world will be a healthier and more beautiful place because of your efforts.

Appendix

Here is the complete Energetic Constitution Survey referred to in chapter 1 along with instructions on how to tally your numerical score and with a patient example to better illustrate how the calculations work. Again, note that this form lives on my website at www.jdyangmd.com so you can reevaluate your energetic status throughout the year as necessary.

YANG DEFICIENCY

QUESTIONS	NEVER	OCCASIONALLY	SOMETIMES	OFTEN	ALWAYS
1. Do your hands or feet ever feel cold?	1	2	3	4	5
2. Are your stomach/ abdomen, back, lower back, or knees sensitive to the cold?	1	2	3	4	5
3. Do you wear more clothing than other people to keep warm because you are very sensitive to cold temperatures?	1	2	3	4	5
4. Are you less tolerant of cold temperatures than others? (i.e., less tolerant of the winter, air-conditioning, or fans)?	1	2	3	4	5
5. Are you prone to catching colds more than others or to retaining water in your body?	1	2	3	4	5

Yang Deficiency questionnaire (continued)

QUESTIONS	NEVER	OCCASIONALLY	SOMETIMES	OFTEN	ALWAYS
6. Do you feel uncomfortable when you eat cold food or drink cold beverages? Or do you have an aversion to cold food and beverages?	1	2	3	4	5
7. After you are exposed to the cold or have cold food or beverages, do you tend to develop diarrhea?	1	2	3	4	5

SCORE:_____

YIN DEFICIENCY

QUESTIONS	NEVER	OCCASIONALLY	SOMETIMES	OFTEN	ALWAYS
1. Do you ever feel hot on your palms or on the soles of your feet?	1	2	3	4	5
2. Do your face and body feel feverish?	1	2	3	4	5
3. Do your skin and lips feel dry?	1	2	3	4	5
4. Are your lips naturally redder than others' lips?	1	2	3	4	5
5. Are you easily constipated or do you have dry stools?	1	2	3	4	5
6. Is your face flushed or reddish in color?	1	2	3	4	5
7. Do you have a dry mouth or dry eyes?	1	2	3	4	5
8. Do you sweat easily upon mild exertion, or do you sweat at night?	1	2	3	4	5

SCORE:_____

QI DEFICIENCY

Questions	Never	Occasionally	Sometimes	Often	Always
1. Are you easily tired?	1	2	3	4	5
2. Do you experience shortness of breath or have difficulty catching your breath?	1	2	3	4	5
3. Do you get heart palpitations easily?	1	2	3	4	5
4. Do you get light-headed or dizzy when you stand up?	1	2	3	4	5
5. Do you catch cold more often than others?	1	2	3	4	5
6. Do you prefer being silent to talking?	1	2	3	4	5
7. Is your voice weak when you are speaking?	1	2	3	4	5
8. Do you sweat spontaneously or with only mild exertion?	1	2	3	4	5

SCORE:_____

DAMPNESS AND PHLEGM

Questions	Never	Occasionally	Sometimes	Often	Always
1. Do you feel congestion in your chest and are you bloated or full in your abdominal region?	1	2	3	4	5
2. Do you feel heaviness throughout your entire body and limbs?	1	2	3	4	5
3. Do you have a lot of belly fat?	1	2	3	4	5

Dampness and Phlegm questionnaire (*continued*)

QUESTIONS	NEVER	OCCASIONALLY	SOMETIMES	OFTEN	ALWAYS
4. Do you have an oily secretion on your forehead?	1	2	3	4	5
5. Are your upper eyelids swollen?	1	2	3	4	5
6. Do you have a sticky feeling in your mouth?	1	2	3	4	5
7. Do you have a lot of phlegm, and does it always make you feel as if your throat is being blocked?	1	2	3	4	5
8. Do you have a thick, greasy coating on your tongue?	1	2	3	4	5

SCORE:_____

DAMPNESS AND HEAT

QUESTIONS	NEVER	OCCASIONALLY	SOMETIMES	OFTEN	ALWAYS
1. Do your face and nose feel greasy or look luminous due to excessive oil secretion?	1	2	3	4	5
2. Do you develop acne and boils easily?	1	2	3	4	5
3. Do you have a bitter or other peculiar taste in your mouth?	1	2	3	4	5
4. Do you feel as if your stool is sticky and hard to eliminate completely?	1	2	3	4	5
5. Do you have a burning sensation when you urinate? Is your urine a dark yellow color?	1	2	3	4	5

Questions	Never	Occasionally	Sometimes	Often	Always
6. For women: Is your vaginal discharge a yellow color?	1	2	3	4	5
7. For men: Do you feel wet or damp on your scrotum?	1	2	3	4	5

Score:_____

BLOOD STASIS

Questions	Never	Occasionally	Sometimes	Often	Always
1. Do you have signs of purple petechia (bleeding under the skin)?	1	2	3	4	5
2. Do you have visible capillaries on your cheeks?	1	2	3	4	5
3. Do you have pain anywhere on your body?	1	2	3	4	5
4. Does your facial coloring appear dark or gloomy? Are you prone to having chloasma (dark brown spots) on your face?	1	2	3	4	5
5. Are you prone to having black circles around your eyes?	1	2	3	4	5
6. Do you tend to be forgetful?	1	2	3	4	5
7. Is your natural lip color purplish?	1	2	3	4	5

Score:_____

SENSITIVITIES

Questions	Never	Occasionally	Sometimes	Often	Always
1. Do you sneeze even when you do not have a cold?	1	2	3	4	5
2. Do you have nasal congestion and a runny nose even when you do not have a cold?	1	2	3	4	5
3. Do you cough or wheeze in reaction to the change of seasons and climate or in reaction to fragrances?	1	2	3	4	5
4. Do you tend to be allergic to medicines, foods, odors, pollen, or season and climate changes?	1	2	3	4	5
5. Do you have urticaria (hives or raised light red bumps) on your skin?	1	2	3	4	5
6. Do you have purpura (purplish red discoloration) on your skin due to allergies?	1	2	3	4	5
7. Does your skin look scraped when you scratch it?	1	2	3	4	5

SCORE:_____

QI STAGNATION

Questions	Never	Occasionally	Sometimes	Often	Always
1. Do you feel unhappy?	1	2	3	4	5
2. Do you easily feel nervous or anxious?	1	2	3	4	5
3. Are you overly sentimental and emotionally fragile?	1	2	3	4	5
4. Do you feel scared or frightened?	1	2	3	4	5

Questions	Never	Occasionally	Sometimes	Often	Always
5. Do you have congestion or pain in your breast or hypochondriac area (the region just above your abdomen)?	1	2	3	4	5
6. Do you sigh for no apparent reason?	1	2	3	4	5
7. Do you feel something in your throat that you cannot spit up?	1	2	3	4	5

SCORE:_____

BALANCED Q*I*

Questions	Never	Occasionally	Sometimes	Often	Always
1. Are you energetic?	1	2	3	4	5
2. Are you prone to feeling fatigued?	5	4	3	2	1
3. Is your voice weak when you are speaking?	5	4	3	2	1
4. Do you feel unhappy?	5	4	3	2	1
5. Is your body more sensitive to cold temperatures than others (i.e., sensitive to the winter, air-conditioning, or fans)?	5	4	3	2	1
6. Do you adapt well to changes in natural or social environments?	1	2	3	4	5
7. Do you have insomnia?	5	4	3	2	1
8. Are you forgetful?	5	4	3	2	1

SCORE:_____

NAME:_____ **DATE:**_____

HOW TO TALLY THE RESULTS

If you've completed the questionnaire on pages 227 through 233, the following steps will help you arrive at a more accurate assessment than the self-assessment you practiced earlier on pages 8 through 12. Note that each set of questions must be scored *separately* as follows:

1. Tally the numbers associated with your answers in each section. That total will become your "original score."
2. Subtract the number of questions in the section (there will be seven or eight) from your original score and set that number aside.
3. Then multiply the number of questions in the section by four and divide the answer from step 2 of this list by this product.
4. Now multiply by 100 and you will have your final score for that portion of the questionnaire.
5. The formula should look like this: **(Original score – Number of questions) ÷ (Number of questions x 4) x 100 = Final score**

If the score for the set of questions measuring your *Qi* Balance (the last set of questions) is equal to or greater than 60 and the score for all of the other sections is equal to or less than 30, consider yourself well balanced!

If the score for the set of questions measuring your *Qi* Balance is equal to or greater than 60 and the score for all of the other sections is equal to or less than 40, consider yourself generally balanced.

If any of the sets of questions are not meeting the criteria set here—if the *Qi* Balance score is below 60 or any of the other scores are above 40—then the energy that particular set of questions is designed to evaluate is very likely in need of balancing.

SAMPLE QUESTIONNAIRE COMPLETED BY A FIFTY-YEAR-OLD PATIENT NAMED KAY

YANG DEFICIENCY

QUESTIONS	NEVER	OCCASIONALLY	SOMETIMES	OFTEN	ALWAYS
1. Do your hands or feet ever feel cold?	1	2 X	3	4	5
2. Are your stomach/ abdomen, back, lower back, or knees sensitive to the cold?	1 X	2	3	4	5
3. Do you wear more clothing than other people to keep warm because you are very sensitive to cold temperatures?	1	2 X	3	4	5
4. Are you less tolerant of cold temperatures than others? (i.e., less tolerant of the winter, air-conditioning, or fans)?	1	2 X	3	4	5
5. Are you prone to catching colds more than others or to retaining water in your body?	1	2	3 X	4	5
6. Do you feel uncomfortable when you eat cold food or drink cold beverages? Or do you have an aversion to cold food and beverages?	1	2 X	3	4	5
7. After you are exposed to the cold or have cold food or beverages, do you tend to develop diarrhea?	1	2 X	3	4	5

SCORE: 25

Formula: (Original score – Number of questions) ÷ (Number of questions x 4) x 100

In Kay's case: (14 – 7) ÷ (7 x 4) x 100 = (7 ÷ 28) x 100 = 25

YIN DEFICIENCY

Questions	Never	Occasionally	Sometimes	Often	Always
1. Do you ever feel hot on your palms or on the soles of your feet?	1	2	3 X	4	5
2. Do your face and body feel feverish?	1	2	3 X	4	5
3. Do your skin and lips feel dry?	1	2	3 X	4	5
4. Are your lips naturally redder than others' lips?	1	2 X	3	4	5
5. Are you easily constipated or do you have dry stools?	1	2	3 X	4	5
6. Is your face flushed or reddish in color?	1	2	3 X	4	5
7. Do you have a dry mouth or dry eyes?	1	2 X	3	4	5
8. Do you sweat easily upon mild exertion, or do you sweat at night?	1	2 X	3	4	5

SCORE: 40.6

Score = (21 – 8) ÷ (8 x 4) x 100 = (13 ÷ 32) x 100 = 40.6

QI DEFICIENCY

Questions	Never	Occasionally	Sometimes	Often	Always
1. Are you easily tired?	1	2	3 X	4	5
2. Do you experience shortness of breath or have difficulty catching your breath?	1	2	3 X	4	5
3. Do you get heart palpitations easily?	1	2	3 X	4	5
4. Do you get light-headed or dizzy when you stand up?	1	2	3 X	4	5

QUESTIONS	NEVER	OCCASIONALLY	SOMETIMES	OFTEN	ALWAYS
5. Do you catch cold more often than others?	1	2	3 X	4	5
6. Do you prefer being silent to talking?	1	2 X	3	4	5
7. Is your voice weak when you are speaking?	1	2 X	3	4	5
8. Do you sweat spontaneously or with only mild exertion?	1 X	2	3	4	5

SCORE: 37.5

Score = (20 – 8) ÷ (8 x 4) x 100 = (12 ÷ 32) x 100 = 37.5

DAMPNESS AND PHLEGM

QUESTIONS	NEVER	OCCASIONALLY	SOMETIMES	OFTEN	ALWAYS
1. Do you feel congestion in your chest and are you bloated or full in your abdominal region?	1	2	3 X	4	5
2. Do you feel heaviness throughout your entire body and limbs?	1	2 X	3	4	5
3. Do you have a lot of belly fat?	1	2	3	4	5 X
4. Do you have an oily secretion on your forehead?	1 X	2	3	4	5
5. Are your upper eyelids swollen?	1 X	2	3	4	5
6. Do you have a sticky feeling in your mouth?	1 X	2	3	4	5

Dampness and Phlegm questionnaire *(continued)*

Questions	Never	Occasionally	Sometimes	Often	Always
7. Do you have a lot of phlegm, and does it always make you feel as if your throat is being blocked?	1	2 X	3	4	5
8. Do you have a thick, greasy coating on your tongue?	1 X	2	3	4	5

SCORE: 25

Score = (16 – 8) ÷ (8 x 4) x 100 = (8 ÷ 32) x 100 = 25

DAMPNESS AND HEAT

Questions	Never	Occasionally	Sometimes	Often	Always
1. Do your face and nose feel greasy or look luminous due to excessive oil secretion?	1 X	2	3	4	5
2. Do you develop acne and boils easily?	1 X	2	3	4	5
3. Do you have a bitter or other peculiar taste in your mouth?	1	2 X	3	4	5
4. Do you feel as if your stool is sticky and hard to eliminate completely?	1	2 X	3	4	5
5. Do you have a burning sensation when you urinate? Is your urine a dark yellow color?	1	2 X	3	4	5
6. For women: Is your vaginal discharge a yellow color?	1	2 X	3	4	5
7. For men: Do you feel wet or damp on your scrotum?	1	2	3	4	5

SCORE: 16.6

Score = (10 – 6) ÷ (6 x 4) x 100 = (4 ÷ 24) x 100 = 16.6

BLOOD STASIS

Questions	Never	Occasionally	Sometimes	Often	Always
1. Do you have signs of purple petechia (bleeding under the skin)?	1 X	2	3	4	5
2. Do you have visible capillaries on your cheeks?	1 X	2	3	4	5
3. Do you have pain anywhere on your body?	1	2	3 X	4	5
4. Does your facial coloring appear dark or gloomy? Are you prone to having chloasma (dark brown spots) on your face?	1 X	2	3	4	5
5. Are you prone to having black circles around your eyes?	1 X	2	3	4	5
6. Do you tend to be forgetful?	1	2	3 X	4	5
7. Is your natural lip color purplish?	1	2 X	3	4	5

SCORE: 17.85

Score = (12 – 7) ÷ (7 x 4) x 100 = (5 ÷ 28) x 100 = 17.85

SENSITIVITIES

Questions	Never	Occasionally	Sometimes	Often	Always
1. Do you sneeze even when you do not have a cold?	1	2	3	4 X	5
2. Do you have nasal congestion and a runny nose even when you do not have a cold?	1	2	3	4 X	5
3. Do you cough or wheeze in reaction to the change of seasons and climate or in reaction to fragrances?	1	2	3	4 X	5

Sensitivities questionnaire *(continued)*

QUESTIONS	NEVER	OCCASIONALLY	SOMETIMES	OFTEN	ALWAYS
4. Do you tend to be allergic to medicines, foods, odors, pollen, or season and climate changes?	1	2	3	4 X	5
5. Do you have urticaria (hives or raised light red bumps) on your skin?	1	2	3 X	4	5
6. Do you have purpura (purplish red discoloration) on your skin due to allergies?	1	2 X	3	4	5
7. Does your skin look scraped when you scratch it?	1 X	2	3	4	5

SCORE: 53.57

Score = (22 – 7) ÷ (7 x 4) x 100 = (15 ÷ 28) x 100 = 53.57

QI STAGNATION

QUESTIONS	NEVER	OCCASIONALLY	SOMETIMES	OFTEN	ALWAYS
1. Do you feel unhappy?	1	2	3 X	4	5
2. Do you easily feel nervous or anxious?	1	2	3	4 X	5
3. Are you overly sentimental and emotionally fragile?	1	2	3 X	4	5
4. Do you feel scared or frightened?	1	2	3 X	4	5
5. Do you have congestion or pain in your breast or hypochondriac area (the region just above your abdomen)?	1	2	3	4 X	5

QUESTIONS	NEVER	OCCASIONALLY	SOMETIMES	OFTEN	ALWAYS
6. Do you sigh for no apparent reason?	1	2	3 X	4	5
7. Do you feel something in your throat that you cannot spit up?	1	2	3 X	4	5

SCORE: 57.14

Score = (23 – 7) ÷ (7 x 4) x 100 = (16 ÷ 28) x 100 = 57.14

BALANCED QI

QUESTIONS	NEVER	OCCASIONALLY	SOMETIMES	OFTEN	ALWAYS
1. Are you energetic?	1	2	3 X	4	5
2. Are you prone to feeling fatigued?	5	4	3 X	2	1
3. Is your voice weak when you are speaking?	5	4 X	3	2	1
4. Do you feel unhappy?	5	4	3 X	2	1
5. Is your body more sensitive to cold temperatures than others (i.e., sensitive to the winter, air-conditioning, or fans)?	5	4 X	3	2	1
6. Do you adapt well to changes in natural or social environments?	1	2	3	4 X	5
7. Do you have insomnia?	5	4 X	3	2	1
8. Are you forgetful?	5	4	3 X	2	1

SCORE: 62.5

Score = (28 – 8) ÷ (8 x 4) x 100 = (20 ÷ 32) x 100 = 62.5

Name: Kay   Date: June 2015

You will note that two of Kay's scores were much higher than the targeted range—the ones measuring *Qi* Stagnation and Sensitivities. This indicates that the flow of her energies may be blocked or misdirected, impeding the normal function of the whole system. The proper flow of energy needs to be restored and better balanced in these areas.

In addition, her *Qi* is also overly sensitive to environmental energy. This is often due to an underlying *Qi* Deficiency in the Lungs. She needs to be desensitized and replenished with *Qi* in her Lungs.

How did you score?

"Chinese Medicine Questionnaire on Physical Constitution" designed under the leadership of Professor Qi Wang, tenure professor and grandmaster of Chinese medicine, Beijing University of Chinese Medicine.

THE TWELVE MAJOR MERIDIANS

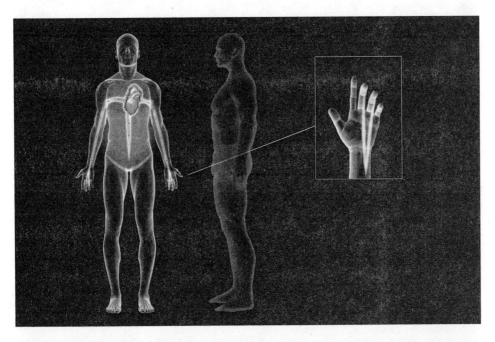

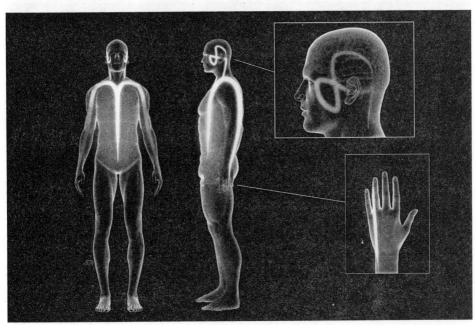

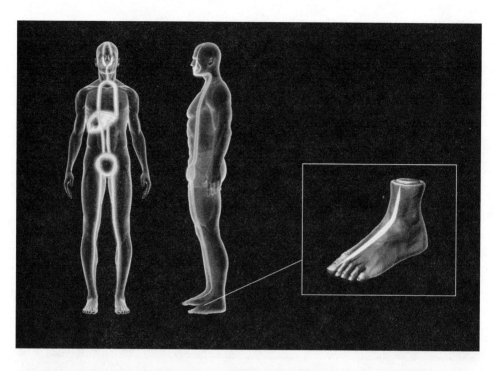

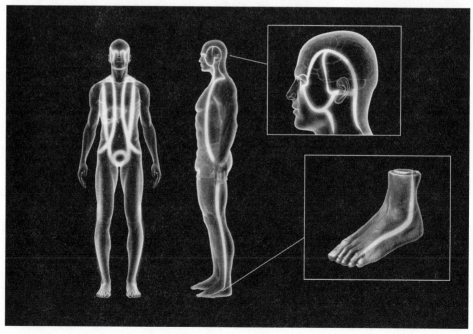

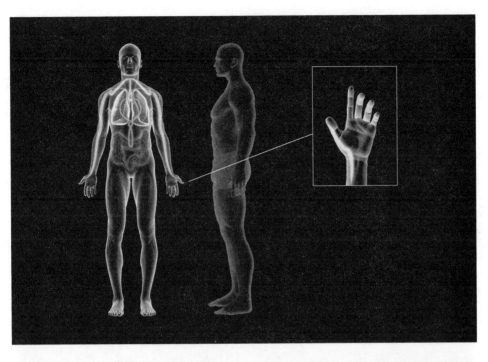

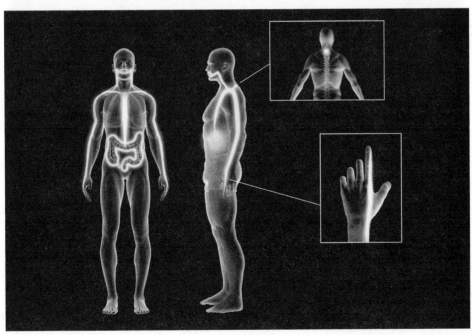

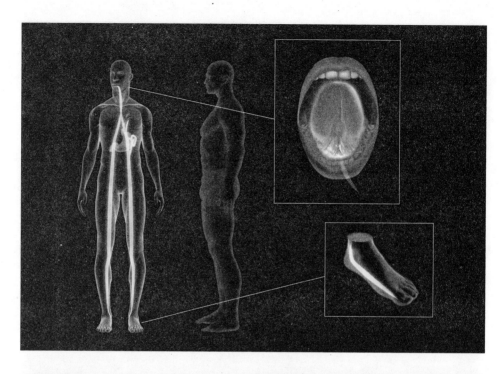

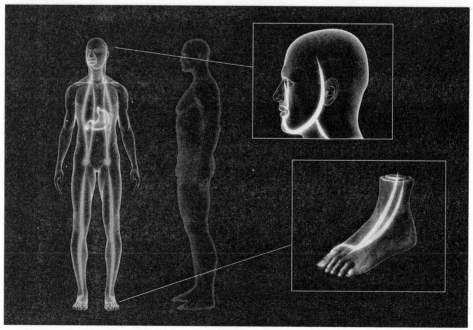

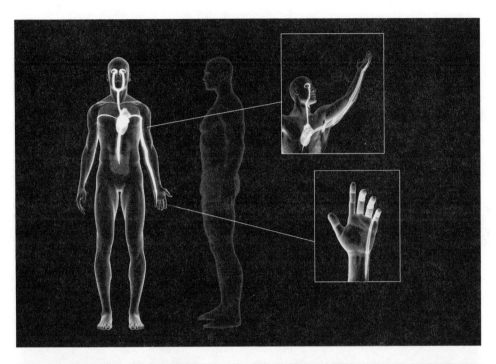

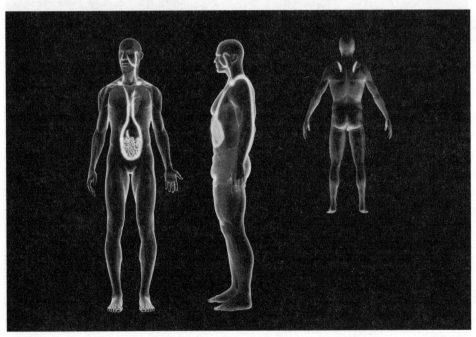

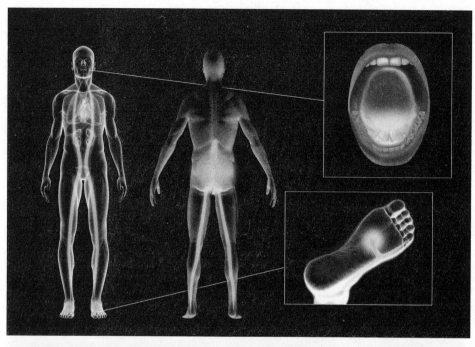

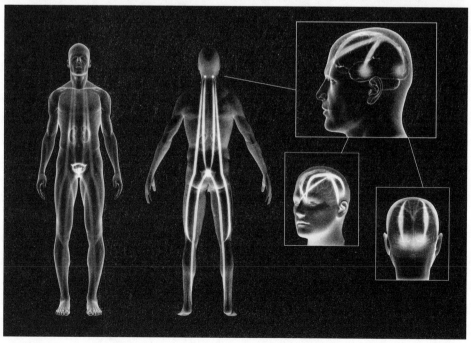

About the Authors

JINGDUAN YANG, M.D., F.A.P.A.

Dr. Jingduan Yang is a leading physician, board-certified psychiatrist, and international expert on classical forms of Chinese medicine. He uniquely incorporates acupuncture, Chinese herbal medicine, neuro-emotional technique, nutritional and dietary consultation, psychotherapy, and medication management in the care of patients with a variety of physical and emotional illnesses.

Following family tradition, he is a fifth-generation teacher and practitioner of Chinese medicine, specializing in acupuncture. Dr. Yang received his medical and neurology training at the Fourth Military Medical University in Xian, China, where he studied with the renowned Dr. Guoxiong You. As one of the first students to study outside of China on an exchange program with the University of Sydney in Australia, he also had the distinct honor of studying under Professor Thomas Stapleton, M.D., chairman of the Institute of Child Health, and later to complete a research fellowship in clinical psychopharmacology at Oxford University in the United Kingdom with Dr. Philips Cowen and Professor Michael Gelder.

When he relocated to the United States, Dr. Yang worked as a professor at the Minnesota Institute of Acupuncture and Herbal Studies while obtaining all necessary credentialing to be a licensed U.S. physician. He then completed residency training in psychiatry at Thomas Jefferson University in Philadelphia.

Dr. Yang has authored numerous peer-reviewed articles and book chapters in his fields of expertise, and he has been a speaker at several national and international conferences and academic forums. In 2008, awarded with the Bravewell Fellowship, Dr. Yang completed a two-year-long prestigious Integrative Medicine Fellowship at the University of Arizona. This fellowship was launched in 2000 by internationally recognized integrative medicine pioneer Dr. Andrew Weil. Dr. Yang has been a certified neuro-emotional technique practitioner since early 2011. He is also the founder and medical director of the Tao Institute of Mind and Body Medicine.

In addition, Dr. Yang is the director of the Acupuncture and Oriental Medicine Program at the Myrna Brind Center of Integrative Medicine and assistant professor of psychiatry and emergency medicine at the Thomas Jefferson University Hospitals. Dr. Yang is also currently on the faculty of the Center for Integrative Medicine at the University of Arizona. He is a board member of the International Network of Integrative Mental Health and of Mental Health Issues of Diabetes; a fellow of the American Psychiatric Association; and a member of both the American Medical Association and the American Medical Acupuncture Association.

NORMA KAMALI

Norma Kamali is a prolific and iconic designer who has created unforgettable designs and trends: The Sleeping Bag Coat, Farrah Fawcett's Red Swim Suit, and The Parachute Dress. She is known for her innovative yet timeless approach to fashion. Norma's career spans over four decades, and her designs are recognized worldwide. Her clothing is coveted by top celebrities and stylists alike.

Norma Kamali is known not only for her swim collection; her other bodies of work include timeless modern clothing in every classification. Beauty, health, and wellness are clearly woven into her DNA. That DNA, along with her understanding of the human form, sets her apart from all others.

Norma Kamali has won numerous awards for her designs, as well as for her fashion films, architectural designs, and interior designs. Among them is an honorary doctorate from the Fashion Institute of Technology awarded in 2010. She is also the recipient of several Coty Awards and CFDA Awards—including the CFDA Board of Directors' Special Tribute Award, conferred upon her in 2005—as well as a plaque on the Fashion Walk of Fame. Pieces from her collections are included in the Smithsonian National Museum of American History and the Metropolitan Museum of Art. The influence she has had on the fashion industry can be seen throughout her career. Norma has been ahead of the curve in fashion but also in other areas as well. The no makeup, makeup collection in the early 1990s, her fitness line of technical active clothing, and her early use of the Internet in the 1990s to interact directly with her clients are a few examples. Her 3D films, involvement in virtual and augmented reality for education, entertainment, and fashion are all used in a unique way to tell the story of her brand.

After decades of designing, Norma decided to finally reach women who couldn't afford designer clothes, giving them the opportunity to have design, fit, and quality at an amazing price. In 2012, Norma created the collection KAMALI-KULTURE, the next step after her line for Walmart.

The launch of Norma Kamali's SWEATS collection for spring 2014 was a fast-forward look to the future of the revolutionary Sweats collection she originally launched in 1980. That was the first time women wore sweatshirt clothing to work and parties, making one of the first statements about casual clothing. It became a lifestyle movement. The SWEATS collection is another testament to Norma's belief that timeless style is more powerful than fashion, or is in fact real fashion.

At the same time, Norma created and launched ACTIVE, a collection that displays her innate understanding of the contemporary lifestyle of women because she too lives it. This collection springs from Norma's vision of the simplicity of fitness, health, and beauty merging together, and bound by the sophistication of a designer's point of view. This line is technical activewear but is lifestyle casual with an editorial edge.

Both the SWEATS and ACTIVE collections display Norma's innate understanding of the contemporary lifestyle of women.

In 2001, Norma created the WELLNESS CAFÉ, in New York City, which promotes fitness, health, and alternative beauty solutions. In 2012, she launched her Hey Baby campaign for the empowerment of women. The campaign's mission statement is to bring awareness to the detrimental effects of objectification on women's self-esteem and body image.